Praise for
Bloated?

In our social media, share-it-all, TMI world, most people are still too embarrassed to talk about something we all do: poop and pass gas. In *Bloated?*, Dr. Edison de Mello kicks open the bathroom door and addresses this taboo—and the resulting epidemic of digestive problems—with compassion, concern, and hard-won wisdom. He offers clear, concise answers to the vital question so many of us ask: Why don't I feel better?

—Mark Hyman, MD, *New York Times* Bestselling Author
of *The Pegan Diet*; Head of Strategy—The Cleveland Clinic
Center for Functional Medicine; Founder—The UltraWellness
Center; President, The Institute of Functional Medicine

Edison de Mello is a gifted healer; he can turn a routine annual check-up into a master's class in compassion, biochemistry, and diagnostic insight. With *Bloated?*, he's taken these gifts to the page, offering a smart, helpful and comprehensive look at why so many of us feel so lousy. Blending cutting edge science with personal anecdotes and relatable case histories, Dr. de Mello explores the reasons behind the "bloating epidemic" and offers practical, manageable solutions. So, put down the potato chips, toss out the Tums, stop blaming the dog for the gas you just passed, and pick up *Bloated?*—relief is on the way!

—Roy Sekoff, Founding Editor, *The Huffington Post*

Dr. Edison de Mello has been my primary doctor since 2009. He has guided me in ways that have led to breakthrough after breakthrough in generating robust health. Now, with deep medical understandings and a healthy blend of humor, Dr. de Mello brings much-needed help to BLOATING and Gut Imbalance, little-understood and complex health issues. If you or someone you love suffers from any kind of gut challenges, look no further for answers and easy-to-understand ways for optimizing your Gut so that you can have the health and vitality you've dreamed of. This book can, literally, change your life.

—Mary Morrissey, Founder of Brave Thinking Institute

Dr. Edison de Mello has accomplished an almost impossible feat: writing a well-researched, personal, funny, comforting and incredibly wise book about poop! In three decades of talking to people about their relationship with food, no one has ever mentioned digestion, elimination, or "stink bombs," as Dr. de Mello calls them. Instead, they hide. They feel shame. And they continue to suffer. *Bloated?* changes all that by shining light on the unspoken reasons why people don't ask for help and keep eating foods their bodies don't like and, in the process, offers solutions to vibrant health.

—Geneen Roth, Author of #1 *New York Times* Bestseller, *Women Food and God and This Messy Magnificent Life*

My health has been in the knowledgeable hands of Dr. D. for over a decade, and yet, I constantly learn more from him, especially as I age and my health needs change. Those who don't live in Southern California can now get the benefits of Dr. de Mello's wisdom through his fantastic book. One of the great takeaways for me is Chapter 7, "The Three Amigos": when you think of your gut as a third brain, it's a no-brainer to nourish it to get the right signals to your brain and your heart. This book will add years of vibrant health to your life

—Allison Anders, Filmmaker/Director

The challenge in evaluating the bloated patient involves accounting for the magnitude and diversity of different physiologic errors that end in disruptive intestinal gas. It is so very complex. Yet Dr. De Mello has simplified the method for the layman in this how-to manual on how to reverse bloat. The holy grail of gastroenterology is demystified in this wonderful book. It is told in a light and fresh tone of discovery. Kudos to Dr. De Mello.

—Leo Treyzon, M.D., M.S., Attending Gastroenterologist, Cedars-Sinai Medical Center; Assistant Professor, UCLA Geffen School of Medicine

The Dreschers are overeaters from way back. My mother admitted, "I eat until I'm nauseous, and then I stop . . . usually." My father was finished eating only when he needed to unzip his pants! A humongous belch was a testament of a great meal, and Tums was the after-dinner mint of choice. Needless to say, no family needed Dr. de Mello's book *Bloated?* more than the Dreschers! What a rude awakening it was for my folks to discover they've been eating all wrong and that the post breakfast, lunch and dinner symphony of flatulence was NOT NORMAL! Read the book and get your diet, digestion and defecating on track too! Be HEALTHY for once and for all!

—Fran Drescher, Actress; Author; Founder, Cancer Schmancer Movement

Dr. Edison de Mello is a gifted integrative physician who has effectively summarized his decades-long experience on why people get bloated and how to fix it. Because most people with bloating suffer in silence, often too embarrassed to discuss their symptoms, Dr. de Mello has succeeded in kicking open the bathroom door to discuss the "bloating epidemic" openly and constructively. Utilizing his signature approach of *"meeting his patients before he meets their disease,"* Dr. de Mello has discussed the issue at hand with the deep compassion and wisdom that he is known for while also reminding us that a bit of laughter can be healing. He offers clear and to-the-point answers to the vital question: Why don't I feel better?

—Cynthia Kersey, Best-Selling Author, *Unstoppable*;
Founder & CEO, Unstoppable Foundation

In today's fast-food world where many are eating in ways that are calorically rich and nutritionally poor, attention to diet and gut health has never been more important. If you've ever felt out of sorts (and who hasn't) because of your diet, Dr. Edison de Mello has written a book just for you . . . one that you will find informative, instructive and, perhaps most importantly, enjoyable. I encourage you to get your copy today!

—Blaine Barlett, Best-Selling Author; Teaching Faculty,
American Association for Physician Leadership

What we turn away from will eventually show up in the bowels of our being. We are whole, amazing organisms: mind, body and spirit. In a brilliant and digestible way, Dr. de Mello's book, *Bloated?*, addresses how we can take care of the unconscious way we treat our bodies. I love how he speaks about the consequences of our actions by normalizing talking about something we all do, poop.

—Doriena Wolff, Diamond Approach Teacher

As someone who has made my own health a top priority in recent years, I know firsthand that the food you eat should be a source of healing and not a source of pain, which is why *Bloated?* is a must-read for anyone looking to improve their well-being by learning how to treat their gut. Dr. de Mello offers an easy-to-follow strategy for ensuring that your mindset, and heartset, are aligned with your stomachset.

—David Meltzer, Co-founder of Sports 1 Marketing,
Best-Selling Author, and Top Business Coach

"Hello, Edison, I just got a call. Mom is in the hospital with a diagnosis of acute leukemia and not expected to make it through the night!" This is a typical call I have had with the amazing healer Dr. Edison de Mello over the years. My 76-year-old mother lived to 92 under his loving, skillful guidance. His uncanny insights into people's psychology combined with a wealth of medical knowledge and common-sense wisdom has benefited so many people I know directly, including me. And now, an invaluable gift to us all: he combines his gifts and experience into a funny, clear and comprehensive book, *Bloated?*, addressing our most common digestive issues. A must-read for anyone who is suffering from gas, bloating and other stinky business.

—Reuben Wolff, Psy.D., Clinical Psychologist

An enjoyable and easy-to-read book with clear information and encouragement to anyone suffering from gut conditions driven by gut bacterial overgrowth. Dr. Mello succeeded in presenting the perfect balance of science and warmth mixed with humor to remind us of the healing power of laughter. Just like sitting across from him in his office, his engaging and compassionate bedside manner is easily palpable throughout the book. It is a must-read for another affected by this annoying, embarrassing—and often gut highjacking—disorder.

—Dhru Purohit, CEO, Podcast Host and Entrepreneur

Bloated? is a MUST READ for anyone who's ever experienced any type of abdominal discomfort. It addresses everything you ever wanted to know and explains so much more than you ever imagined about your gut. Dr. Edison de Mello brilliantly explains why so many of us feel so lousy while also offering clear, concise and practical solutions. As an infertility specialist, I know that IVF has a better chance of working if the patient's GI system is well-balanced.

—Shahin Ghadir, MD, F.A.C.O.G., Reproductive Endocrinology and Infertility; Assistant Clinical Professor, UCLA and USC

EDISON DE MELLO, MD, PHD

Foreword by Lee Daniels

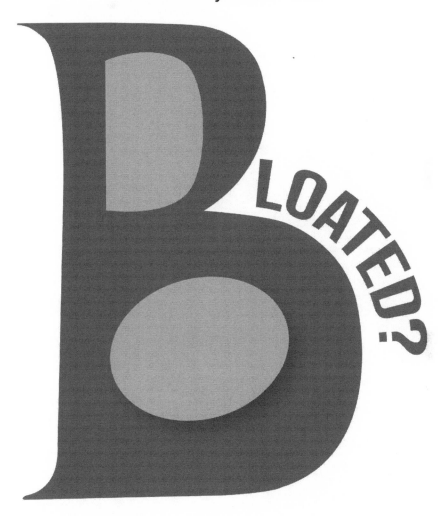

How To Reclaim Your
Gut Health And Eat Without Pain

Published by Elevate Publishing
Cover Concept by Luana Viana

First Edition: June 2021

Library of Congress Control Number: 2021938255

ISBN 978-0-9991949-2-8 (paperback)

Printed in the United States of America

For bulk purchases, contact the publisher at support@elevatebookpublishing.com

To my first integrative medicine teacher—my grandmother, Nana. She's gone now, but her "teachings" are still the foundation of my medical practice.

Contents

Foreword

"Mr. Daniels, with all due respect, it looks like you do not want to be here. So, why are you here? You're free to go at any time. But if you want me to help you, then be *here!*"

And so began my first medical visit with Dr. de Mello. I had been brought to him by a friend who knew that I was, once again, on my self-destructive hamster wheel. I was more than 60 pounds overweight, I had had a recent heart attack, my blood pressure and cholesterol were sky-high, my diet was horrendously bad, and my gut was a mess. I was bloated, fatigued, and my brain was foggy. I was on the verge of becoming diabetic. Death was knocking at my door.

I told Dr. de Mello that I had grown up in a New York City housing project where gun violence and drug deaths were an everyday occurrence. He lovingly—yet decisively—looked me in the eye and said, "You have dodged many bullets in your life and managed to survive, Mr. Daniels. You are a Hollywood icon, an Oscar-nominated director, and the father of two beautiful adult children, correct?"

"Yes, Dr. D," I replied.

"So, Mr. Daniels, why do you keep dodging more and more bullets in your life, as if playing Russian roulette? Do you have a death wish?"

How dare he, I thought! Who is this man who can see right through me? Although Dr. de Mello's office was the last place I wanted to be, I told myself to stick with it. After all, no other doctor before him had confronted me so firmly about my stuff—my death wish and my struggles with accepting love while running my health into the ground. He was right. As a Black man in America, the saddest thing is that I was doing to myself what the world expects of me: self-destructing by slowly killing myself. How could I continue to be the role model to African-American men if I did not look at myself in the mirror and say to myself, "You can do better than this, Lee."

My journey with Dr. de Mello has been like no other. By following his gut heath and the *RESET Program* protocols, I've lost 50 pounds and counting, and committed to my sobriety like never before. I started "listening" to my body. My "firstborn child," as he puts it. Meaning, I am the one who takes care of my body's needs, feeds it, clothes it, and puts it to bed. "Mr. Daniels," Dr. de Mello pressed on, "is it correct to say that you treat your children way better than your body?" He was right again. I, sadly, did take care of almost everyone in my family but me. He taught me that I am my body's father.

I have been on this road with Dr. de Mello by my side for almost seven years. I am more interested in my health, in what I eat, and how I care for my body in a way that I have never been before. As Dr. de Mello calls it, my beehive (gut health) is my barometer that guides me through life. His book, *Bloated?*, not only gives you the knowledge that you need to make a difference in your health, it gives you the tools. The same tools that I have used over these past seven years to change my life and embrace my gut as the "seat of my soul," as de Mello describes it.

I am alive today because Dr. de Mello told me what I need to do to stay alive: look at yourself in the mirror, tell yourself you matter, and that all the bullying, all the pain, all the abuse came out of people's ignorance about accepting that you are not who they expected you to be. You are better. Now you have two options. To believe them and continue to self-destroy—or to show them that they were wrong, and prove that to yourself and the world by becoming the healthiest, most grounded person you can be.

I owe my life to this incredible doctor.

—Lee Daniels
Writer, Producer and Director

Preface

Why Write A Book About . . . Poop?

I have witnessed a staggering number of people suffering from bloating. Look around . . . "bloat" is everywhere. I have seen thousands of patients whose debilitating symptoms have stolen not only their good health, but also their joy of eating, playing, living, and even making love. They represent more than fifty percent of my practice.

That is why I am writing a book about poop.

These patients present with a common denominator: they feel uncomfortable, disgusting, and embarrassed. They are suffering from a common ailment. Everywhere you look, you see people with their gut protruding. Bloating has reached epidemic levels.

Some of my patients report being too embarrassed to date because of the amount of *gas* that they pass every day! I've also had patients, more specifically women, who felt depressed, sick, and lost because their previous doctor told them, "There is nothing wrong with you. The labs are normal. Maybe your bloating is emotional?" In other words, their doctors were implying, *"It's all in your head!"*

If you are having these kinds of health issues, you are not alone. Bloating is an equal-opportunity drag. It can affect anyone and everyone, regardless of race, social or economic background, or status.

One of my most significant and rewarding accomplishments as a physician has been to help patients who suffer from bloating to *get their lives back*, by helping them feel healthy, vital, and sexy again. I am honored to have people from all over the world and from all walks of life come to work with me. I see everyone from celebrities, whose personal appearance and robust health are a mandate, to professionals, to stay-at-home parents, and I am able to show them that there is *a better way to feel better.*

About Me

"I meet my patients before I meet their diseases."
—E. de Mello, MD, PhD

I have written more than fifty papers, book chapters, articles, and blogs related to gut health. I hold three post-graduate degrees, two professional licenses, and have worked at an array of health-care facilities. I have attended two medical schools—one where I completed my science requirements and one where I underwent my clinical rotations. I completed my medical residency in Urban Family Medicine at Albert Einstein College of Medicine at Beth Israel Medical Center, in New York City. I am a member of several professional organizations including the AMA, the Academy of Integrative Health and Medicine (AIHM), the Institute for Functional Medicine (IFM), the American Academy of Family Physicians (AMFP), Physicians for Social Responsibility, Doctors Without Borders, and others.

I'm on several medical advisory boards, including American College for Advancement in Medicine (ACAM), the Unstoppable Foundation, Sunray Peace and Meditation Society, the Midwifery Program in Guatemala, and Open Source Health in Canada.

In 2002, just six months after finishing my residency, I founded the Akasha Center for Integrative Medicine in Santa Monica, California. Akasha is a Sanskrit word that means "an invisible force that binds together the four elements of nature from which our world is derived: air, water, earth, fire." Akasha is that ethereal force that combines all the other elements. The Center is the physical embodiment of my vision and commitment to the practice of integrative medicine, which encompasses the visible as well as the invisible.

My passion in medicine is to help every patient get the best possible results by integrating proven scientific approaches while also drawing together the newest technological advances of traditional Western medicine with the ancient wisdom and healing approaches of the East.

I see people from all walks of life, many of whom have gastrointestinal (GI) symptoms so debilitating that they cannot function at home or work. Why do they travel to meet with me? Because I *listen* to them. Unlike most traditional physicians who check in, ask a few quick questions, and check out, I spend two hours interviewing my patients on their initial visit. Why? Because I want *to meet my patient before I meet their disease.*

I am able to help all of my patients get to the bottom of their bloating symptoms and successfully get rid of them. And now, as an author, it is my intention to give YOU, the reader, this same kind of caring, devotion, and commitment to healing in the format of a book. I invite you to join me on this amazing journey from being *bloated* to feeling your *absolute best*—not just once in a while, but all the time.

Acknowledgments

I wish this section had an unlimited number of pages as the list of people to acknowledge would likely be as big as the book.

Suffice it to say, this is not feasible. So, I start by apologizing to anyone I don't mention here but has been part of my journey. To all of you, THANK YOU!

A million thank yous to the staff and practitioners at the Akasha Center for Integrative Medicine in Santa Monica, California, whose unwavering support has allowed me to reach the stars in a way that I never imagined possible. Thank you specifically to our CEO, Rochelle Richards, and to my business partners, Dr. Maggie Ney, Director of the Women's Clinic, and Mark Meyerdirk, Akasha's loving and dedicated attorney. They are the foundation upon which I get to practice the type of healing medicine that transforms lives. Thank you to my first partner in crime when I opened the Akasha Center, Lisa Feldman-Shinavier, whose determination to see me succeed saw no limit. Lisa believed in me more than I did. She was a tour de force behind my decision to open the Akasha Center.

Thank you to my husband Drew Cartwright de Mello, who wakes up with a "yes, you can" smile on his face and goes to sleep with a look that says, "I knew you could"—even when I doubt myself. Drew has been my unofficial co-resident editor. His love, encouragement, and caretaking give the energy and support that allows me to get out there every day to do what I believe medicine is all about for me. Thank you to our children, Olivia, Tashi, and Lucas, who remind me every day about the healing power of unconditional love.

Thank you to my dear friend, Randy Levinson, who was my rock when I did the unthinkable and uprooted my entire life at age 37 and moved from Los Angeles to go to New York City for residency. Randy's parents, Gwen and Marvin Levinson, bestowed their love, time, and pride in me. Their love sustained me through residency in a city known for always being on the go.

Thank you to my dearest friend, Liz Marx, whose deep love for me allowed her to be brutally honest and say, "Hon, these pages aren't any good. You've got to start from scratch."

And thank you to Reuben Wolff, my "soul brother," and to his late wife, Lief Corroon. They sat me in front of a mirror when I doubted my ability to finish medical school and told me not to get up until I could recognize the doctor looking back at me in the mirror. Their love and friendship guided me to a space where I believed in myself.

Thank you to my brilliant research assistant, Hira Khan. Hira's brilliance was vital in my research for this book. Her intellect and caring personality will make her a phenomenal doctor when she gets into a medical school lucky enough to have her.

Thank you to Liz Irons, my editor, whose primary task was to make sense of what I was attempting to convey on these pages and thank you to the always-ready-to help publisher Cliff Pelloni and his one-of-a-kind team.

Thank you to my spiritual mentor, Dhyani Yahoo, who looked right into my eyes when I doubted being capable of going to medical school and asked me, "Who told you you could not?" As life would have it, venerable Dhyani Ywahoo became one of my strongest supporters and, eventually, my patient.

Last but not least, thank you to my rock, my model of a man, my example of what all fathers should be like, my uncle, Ney Vieira. He has been a strong presence in my life for as long as I can remember. Uncle Ney looked shocked when my 15-year-old self asked him if he'd get me a meeting with his boss, Ricardo Marinho, one of the owners of the biggest and most prominent newspaper in Brazil. Mr. Marinho was on the board of Cultura Inglesa, a very expensive and highly regarded English as a Second Language school in my hometown, Rio de Janeiro, Brazil. I wanted to ask Mr. Marinho for a discount on my courses at Cultura Inglesa so that I could better prepare to take an ESL entrance examination that would allow me to qualify for a scholarship to go to college in the United States. My uncle, although a bit shocked at my request, did not hesitate. "Well," he said, "if that's what it is going to take, then count on me." I became more proficient in English, did very well on the entrance examination—and qualified for a scholarship to go to college. I owe this moment to Uncle Ney.

Introduction

*"The microbiome (bacteria balance) is to good health
what a healthy beehive is to good honey."*
—E. de Mello, MD, PhD

Fasten your seat belts because you are about to learn more
about bloating, pooping, and farting than you ever would
have imagined. Maybe more than you thought you wanted to
know. But this book is also about so much more than that. It's
about *why* you are bloated, gassy, fatigued, moody, feeling un-
sexy, or, worst-case scenario, feeling that your life is spinning out
of control! This is a book about something each of our bodies
must do but that we hardly ever talk about: Poop!

We all poop, fart ("pass wind," if you are the Queen of
England), and belch. Research shows that humans fart 14 times a
day, on average. This does for the human body what an exhaust
pipe does for a car. The waste must be eliminated in order for
the engine to work properly.

I want to challenge the myth that talking about bloating and
passing gas is "too embarrassing," or "too personal," or "not
cool." Isn't it interesting that some of us have no qualms about
cleaning our cat's litter box or picking up after our dog's business? And what about changing our baby's diapers, wiping the

mess off their bottoms? But when it comes to talking about our own bloated bellies, passing gas, and irregular poop habits, it's taboo. This does not have to be! The more comfortable you become talking about these uncomfortable issues, the easier it is to overcome them.

Bloating is so common these days that it can actually be referred to as an "epidemic." You hear friends and family complaining that they feel awful. They are upset that their symptoms have taken over their lives. The reasons are multifactorial:

- Poor diets
- Our "eat-on-the-go" culture
- High levels of stress
- Overuse of antibiotics
- Mass production of food
- Exposure to various pollutants in the air, food, and water
- Our unhealthy relationship with food

Each of these factors contribute to our current culture of gut *DIS-ease.*

When Bloating Is a Constant, Uninvited, Annoying Companion

*"Bloating is the language your gut uses to say
this stuff ain't good for us."*

—Edison de Mello, MD, PhD

When I think about it, I realize my own interest in stomach issues started a long time ago when I was growing up in Brazil. My childhood home was very close to the City of God, a notoriously violent housing project in Rio de Janeiro, depicted in the movie of the same name. I still have haunting memories of walking home from school, the sound of gunshots making me feel so scared and vulnerable.

I'd finally get home, yank open the front door and run to the bathroom, which, instead of a solid door, had only a curtain hanging in the door frame. I was incredibly embarrassed that my mom and siblings could hear me passing gas, among other things. My already fragile, 12-year-old self sat there thinking, *"What's wrong with me?* Why can't I just be normal?" It really didn't help that I also suffered from asthma, which was exacerbated when I felt stress.

Because of this, at an early age, I developed a keen interest in how our bodies work, but I had no educational role models in my family. Both of my parents were uneducated. No one in my family had ever finished high school, let alone gone to college. So, I knew I had to look elsewhere for guidance. It was my good fortune that I had an inspiration right in front of me in Nana, my beloved grandmother.

Nana had never set foot in a classroom and was technically illiterate, but she was the smartest, kindest person I knew. She still is, even though she's been gone now for almost thirty years. Nana was the first person to introduce me to the practice of *complementary medicine*. She was a natural healer who, with her many teas and potions, always had a remedy for any common, everyday malady. Nana practiced her "medicine" with so much love and dedication that just her presence—her caring manner, smile, and unwavering respect for people—was healing and inspiring for everyone whose life she touched.

As I got older, my own symptoms persisted and so did my fascination with natural medications. Nana's approach to healing and her loving mentorship were so profound that, when I entered college in the United States, a career in healthcare already felt like a natural choice. I was sending money home to help my struggling mother. My father had left long ago, which was financially challenging for us. The cost of medical school was beyond what I could afford, so I put medicine aside and enrolled in a psychology training program. I graduated with a bachelor's degree in psychology, went on to earn a master's degree in psychology, and then a doctoral degree in health and human services with a focus on psychology.

For my master's thesis, I co-authored a grant for a Head Start program in the San Fernando Valley of Los Angeles, funded by the National Institute of Mental Health, entitled *Strengthening Head Start Families through Mental Health Intervention*.

Following graduation, I was hungry to learn how our bodies talk to us. I wanted to know why I had such intense "gut feelings" when I was a child. I knew the answer resided somewhere in the power of our minds.

It was during research for my Ph.D. dissertation that my calling for medicine resurfaced. I decided that my research topic and title would be *Gut Feelings—A Psychosocial Approach to Gastrointestinal Illness*. I chose Highland Hospital in Oakland, California, as my research site because it provided medical care to people from all over the world.

I began vigorously exploring some very complex gastrointestinal cases where practitioners were struggling to find any medical (pathological) explanations for their patients' conditions. In most cases, when no mental or physical reasons for the symptoms could be found, the *idiopathic* explanation was applied. The term "idiopathic" has the Greek root *pathos*, which means suffering of "unknown cause." It's used frequently in medicine when doctors cannot identify the cause of a particular condition.

I joked with a few doctors on staff that when it comes to understanding the mind-body connection, to use the term "idiopathic" is to say that *we*, the practitioners, are a bunch of idiots. We do not have a clue about the powerful connection between our minds and bodies.

We were seeing a condition that was causing a domino-like effect in the body, disrupting every single organ system: cardiovascular, pulmonary, neurological, and sexual. There were several cases where a patient's GI symptoms were so severe that surgeons scheduled "exploratory abdominal surgery" as a last resort, only to end up at the very place they were before the surgery: a big, fat nowhere.

I became obsessed with the idea of figuring it out, devouring everything I could get my hands on about GI pain and microbial imbalance (dysbiosis). I was completely intrigued by the amazing and complex function of the GI system.

Traditional Chinese Medicine, or TCM, refers to the gut as the "second brain." The biopsychosocial aspects of gastrointestinal disease and the power of the mind were becoming apparent to me. That decades-old feeling resurfaced. I was sure my mission here on this planet was to be a doctor! My nana had seen my vocation even before I did.

After many trials and tribulations, in 1991, I entered medical school. My ultimate goal was to create an innovative medical center that would bridge the gap between Western and Eastern medicines. I envisioned it as a healing sanctuary where all the parts that compose a person—mind, body, and spirit—are addressed equally.

For me, a patient is so much more than just a set of symptoms. He or she is a whole person, experiencing the many trials and tribulations of life. I want to hear about their experiences to see how they might correlate with their "DIS-ease." I will often ask my patients, "If your disease had a message for you, what would that be?"

I want to know more about who they are. What else is going on in their lives besides their diseases? Are they married or single? Are they a mother or father? What is their passion? Do they have a spiritual practice or a pet that helps them with stress? Are they happy with where they are in their lives?

I ask about their intuition, that *inner knowing* of what their bodies are trying to communicate. I impress upon each person that the body is akin to a firstborn child. Who puts your body to sleep, feeds it, and protects it from being hit by a car? You do!

You are your *body's* mama or papa. Are you taking care of your "firstborn"? Are you *listening* to it, paying attention to its symptoms? Are you careful not to put anything into it that your intuition says is not good for it?

An impressive body of recent research has found that certain bacteria in the gut can even affect people's mental state, leading to mood, cognition, and behavioral problems. Traditional Chinese medicine recognized the link between the gut, the brain, and all of the body's organs over five thousand years ago. This second brain, which has also been described in today's medicine as "the little brain," is anything but little.

We have language for this intuition, too. Having a "gut reaction" indicates an innate, inner knowing. Or, you might say you have "butterflies in your stomach" when you feel nervous.

These phrases describe physical signals from the "second brain"—the gut.

This second brain, the Enteric Nervous System (ENS), is composed of two thin layers, each with more than one hundred million nerve cells lining the gastrointestinal tract from esophagus to rectum. Hidden in the walls of the digestive system, this brain-gut connection has become the darling of modern medicine.

Bloating: What the Heck Is It?

Bloating, when the gastrointestinal (GI) tract is filled with excess air or gas, can occur in people of all ages. A person experiencing bloating usually describes their abdomen as feeling "full" or "tight" or "swollen."

This is often accompanied by:

- abdominal pain
- excessive gas (flatulence, farting)
- frequent burping or belching
- abdominal rumbling or gurgles

Abdominal bloating can interfere with your ability to work and participate in social or recreational activities. According to a University of North Carolina study,[1] people who experience abdominal bloating use more sick days, visit the doctor more often, and take more medications than other people. Bloating affects people of all ages, including children.

Why Do You Feel Bloated?

Plain old *gas* is the most common cause of bloating, especially when it happens after eating. Gas builds up in the digestive tract when undigested food leaves the stomach and is broken down in the colon by bacteria, or *flora*. And everyone swallows some air when they eat or drink. But some people consume more, especially if they are eating or drinking too fast, chewing gum, smoking, or wearing loose dentures—yes, really.

Gassiness and abdominal discomfort aren't limited to the occasional holiday extravaganza. A majority of people have experienced some bloating in their lives. It is estimated that at least one in ten Americans suffer from bloating on a regular basis, even when they haven't eaten a large meal.

How Does It *Feel* to Be Bloated?

BALLOON ANALOGY
Doctor, it feels like I swallowed a balloon . . .

A disorder of motility and dysregulation of the central nervous system (CNS), bloating is the most common gastrointestinal disorder that I see in my practice. As a doctor of integrative medicine, my understanding of bloating has evolved from thinking of it as simply excessive abdominal gas to seeing it as a more complex set of markers of one's general health and well-being.

A number of my patients use words like, "swelling," "inflammation," or "feeling pregnant" to describe their symptoms. By describing a balloon-like sensation, they have painted a precise picture of how they feel.

Bloating can be a sign of more complicated disorders like gut bacterial dysbiosis (imbalance), excretion (gut motility), and/or hypersensitivity to certain foods and associated toxins that lead to brain-gut dysfunction.

The description of having the sensation of a balloon inflating in their bellies (bloating), or an increase in their abdominal girth (distension), or sometimes both, is an essential factor in determining if their problem is medical in nature.

Most of my patients who present with symptoms of bloating, say that their bellies puff out, sometimes immediately following a meal. And it isn't always after a big meal. Sadly, many doctors still treat this condition like it is psychosomatic. Although psychosocial factors can certainly influence abnormalities in gut motility via the gut-brain axis—the powerful chemical connections between your gut and brain—the condition is not "in the patient's head." Bloating is real. It is embarrassing, annoying, worrisome, and can significantly disrupt one's life.

Is there a Difference Between Bloating and Abdominal Distention?

Yes. And it is significant. Whereas "bloating" is the sensation of abdominal swelling, abdominal *distention* refers to an *actual physical increase in abdominal size*. With distention, the abdomen is consistently protruding, which may indicate a mass-occupying lesion or a number of other diagnostic possibilities. It should be noted that abdominal distention can actually be a sign of a serious condition. So, while a bloated stomach is uncomfortable, your big gut could also be an indicator of a significant medical issue. For example, bloating is one of the most common symptoms of Candida, IBD (inflammatory bowel disease), SIBO (small intestinal bacterial overgrowth), or even more threatening conditions. It is not something you should let go, unchecked.

One of the most effective steps in attempting to explain what is happening to your body and why is to keep track of exactly what triggers your symptoms.

Given most people's poor diets, high levels of stress, needs for daily medication, and inadvertent exposure to various pollutants, it's no surprise that so many people are suffering from bloating. The most commonly reported symptom is a sensation that the abdomen is "full." If there is pain, it is generally described as "sharp" and, at times, causing the stomach to go into spasms or cramps. And these pains might change locations quickly.

Another common symptom of gas is hiccups. They are generally harmless and will usually diminish on their own, but they can take a long time to resolve and can be very uncomfortable.

People suffering from bloating can help their practitioners arrive at possible causes by accurately and concisely describing their complaints. The more detailed information you can provide, the more you'll help your practitioner arrive at the answers to your questions.

CASE STUDY

Debbie: The "Unseen" Patient

A few years back, I was at a hospital teaching medical residents how to interview patients effectively. It was organized as a hands-on experience, where a real patient was brought in to be interviewed by a resident while the rest of us looked on.

The first patient, "Debbie," was in her mid-forties and had a protruding belly. She looked uncomfortable, had terrible acne, and wore a sad look on her face as if she was in constant pain. She also appeared to be shy, or perhaps she was just embarrassed about her condition.

The resident, whom I shall call "Paul," started the interview. He didn't look directly at her or make eye contact. (Sound familiar?) Nor did he introduce any of us in the room or explain why we were there. Instead, Paul sounded rushed.

It was as if he was late for a more important meeting. He actually blurted out, "Are you pregnant?"

"What?" Debbie recoiled. "No, doctor!"

Then the flood gates opened. "I've had this condition for months and not one single doctor has been able to help me! They can't figure it out, so they tell me to lose weight, or exercise, or they just act like I might be a hypochondriac. And worst of all, like you just did, they take a quick look at me and ask, 'Are you pregnant?' I am *not* pregnant!" she asserted. "Do any of you even have a *clue* what you're doing?"

Welcome to today's practice of medicine.

I took over the interview to show Paul and the other residents how a patient assessment should be done in order to get to a diagnosis. First, I introduced myself and the rest of the team. I thanked Debbie for volunteering to come in so that we could all learn from her experience. Our ultimate goal was to help her and other patients suffering from this painful condition.

Next, I asked where she lived and how her drive to the hospital was. I told her I liked the color of her hair. She relaxed a little, and for the first time since she had walked into the room, Debbie actually smiled.

Then I asked her, "Do you have an *intuition* as to why you're in this pain?"

"Well, I know that I've been dealing with this swelling for three years," Debbie said, placing her hands on her belly. "I have seen five gastroenterologists and another half-dozen internists, and all they say is to take antacids and to stop overeating!" She stamped her foot down. "I DO NOT overeat!"

She continued. "Sometimes they have even said maybe I should seek psychological counseling." Debbie let out a heavy sigh. "In other words, in the end, they think it's all in my head!"

I smiled and asked, "Did anyone ever ask you to do a stool or breath test? Or did they try to rule out an *overgrowth of bacteria*? Did any one of your doctors suggest you try an *elimination diet* to see which foods trigger issues for you?"

"No," she shook her head in surprise, "I do not even know what those things are!"

An Aside on Food Intolerance:
Bloating and gas can often result from food intolerance. An *elimination diet* implemented under the supervision of an integrative healthcare practitioner is the best litmus test to identify which foods your GI system has difficulty tolerating. I often recommend doing an elimination diet, without taking any supplements that alleviate bloating, including probiotics, so as not to mask any of the symptoms that you are trying to isolate. This is a good method to, one-by-one, determine problematic foods.

Back to Debbie . . .
I delivered my prognosis. "From what you described, Debbie, it sounds like you are suffering from a condition called SIBO, which stands for Small Intestinal Bacterial Overgrowth, which leads to—I'll use layman's terms—significant bloating."

She nodded.

"I'd still like to run the tests I mentioned to confirm the diagnosis," I continued. Debbie nodded again and shifted in her seat.

A breath test revealed that she had extremely high levels of the two main gases that are produced by overgrowth of bacteria in the small intestine: hydrogen and methane. High levels of these gases confirmed a diagnosis of SIBO. Further, a blood test showed that she had severe anemia, caused by iron and B12 deficiencies. Her nutritional assessment also highlighted some other areas of vitamin and mineral deficiency.

Not only did Debbie have extremely high levels of *bad* bacteria in her gut, negatively affecting her metabolic function, but those little critters were also dysregulating her menstrual cycle, decreasing her absorption of B12, and subsequently affecting her overall mood and vitality. In essence, this bacteria was hijacking Debbie's life!

For the last few months, Debbie had been getting her "period" every two weeks—about twice as often as usual. Losing too much blood leads to a loss of many elements essential to good health, including iron. Hence, her severe iron deficiency.

Now, fast forward six months. Debbie showed up in my office, almost unrecognizable. After treating her SIBO, replenishing her nutritional deficiencies and regulating her female hormones, we had put Debbie on an anti-inflammatory diet and an exercise regimen. She had a radiant smile. She'd lost 40 pounds, her skin was clear, and her menstrual cycle had normalized.

Debbie asked me for that original resident's email so she could send him a photo of her new self. She also sent a note:

Dear Dr. Paul,

Here is a photo of the "new" me. I am hopeful, for the sake of all patients, that you've learned that not all protruding bellies mean pregnancy—unless of course, you are an obstetrician. When a person comes in to see you, they need your help, not your judgment.

My Putrid-Smelling, Farting Seatmate

Okay, I know that we all, at one time or another, have had an embarrassing fart or have been next to someone who's having one of those moments. Admit it. I know you have. Here's one of my experiences. It happened on a fully booked flight. As luck would have it, that day I had a middle seat. Soon after takeoff, the guy in the seat next to me by the window started passing gas bombs. I'm talking smelly, putrid farts that smelled like rotten eggs mixed with rotting fish. Get the picture?

At first, I thought, *"Wow! This is disgusting. But poor guy, he's probably so embarrassed. Oh well, it will pass."* But it didn't. He kept on lobbing those stink-bombs every two or three minutes!

After the seatbelt signs were turned off, I asked the woman in the seat on the aisle to please let me out. The look on my face must have said it all because she got up quickly, throwing me a compassionate look. I made a mad dash to the back of the plane, gasping for some much-needed fresh air.

Luckily, it was a short flight.

As we were deplaning, I thought about giving the guy my card with a note saying, "I know what it feels like. I can help." But he bolted out in a hurry, as if he were trying to outrun his own smell.

I have treated countless people who have stunk up many rooms and made people run for their lives. As embarrassing and frustrating as these situations are, there is a way out, and there is nothing to be ashamed of.

What Can Be Done?

Adding to the problem of severe indigestion and *fartitis* (not a technical term, sorry) are a number of negative environmental factors that have, unfortunately, become the norm rather than the exception. The alarming availability of junk food and the resulting poor diets, severe stress, and the overuse of medications, when added to the ongoing and relentless exposure to environmental pollutants, create a recipe for disaster.

Unfortunately, millions of people seem to think bloating is something they just need to "learn to live with." People are discouraged by their symptoms, so many think that there is nothing they can do to relieve them. Do you relate? You may have tried some things, and they haven't worked. Maybe you feel a little helpless. *You can choose not to be condemned by this painful reality.*

There is a way to stop the bloating and its many accompanying symptoms. With certain adjustments to your diet and lifestyle, you will be able to live a comfortable, "bloat-free" life.

Keep reading.

CASE STUDY

Mary: The "Set-Time" Pooper

Mary, a 58-year-old woman, came to me with severe and painful bloating accompanied by constipation. She described this as happening, "most of the time!"

Mary broke into tears in my office when she told me her story: "I have had problems since I was a kid. I feel uncomfortable having a bowel movement in my own home when my adult children are visiting, and I certainly never do it in a public restroom! I feel so embarrassed. The noise is so *loud* from all the gas, and the smell is *super* strong! I am so afraid I'll have a 'situation' that I hardly see my friends anymore."

Before coming to me, Mary had enrolled in a "bowel retraining program" designed to alleviate chronic constipation. The program consisted of setting a specific time every day to sit on the toilet and have a bowel movement.

"It worked somewhat," she told me. "At least I could go

out. But it did absolutely nothing for the gas! I started carry-
ing those travel-size air fresheners to spray around me!"

I smiled because I knew just what she meant. I assured
Mary that she was in good hands. My first step was to order
a battery of tests. These included a take-home three-day
stool test to assess her microbiome (the genetic material of
all the microbes—bacteria, fungi, protozoa, and viruses that
live on and inside the human body), a breath test to rule
out SIBO, a nutritional assessment, and a comprehensive
metabolic analysis. I also ordered another breath test that
would rule out Helicobacter Pylori (H. Pylori), which causes
gastroesophageal ulcers and a slew of symptoms, including
constipation.

Next, I started Mary on a specialized diet and a combination of very effective herbs; the same ones described in
break-through studies by several universities, most nota-
bly Johns Hopkins. I will refer to this going forward as the
"Johns Hopkins protocol." Mary was also treated by our in-
house integrative nutritionist and acupuncturist.

Mary returned two weeks later when all her tests were
back. The tests showed that she had a severe case of SIBO,
the likely result of repeated doses of antibiotics given to her
as a child for ongoing ear infections.

And as an adult, as she described it, antibiotics were still
prescribed for "just about anything. My doctors love to pre-
scribe antibiotics for everything, including a mild cold."

Mary showed significant improvement after a couple of
weeks of following her new herb, diet, and acupuncture
regime. We decided together that it made sense to continue. I have a policy with all of my patients to include them
in the decisions that will affect their health. I provide treatment options with pros and cons, and each patient makes
an informed choice that feels right to them.

Because her test results revealed a significantly unbalanced microbiome with increased fat in her undigested foods, increased inflammatory markers, and an overgrowth of yeast (Candida), Mary agreed with me that it was a good idea to try an antifungal medication.

Four weeks later, Mary was sticking to her diet and exercising (no abdominal crunches), and she reported feeling "at least thirty percent better."

Eight weeks later, she was feeling confident enough to accept an invitation to go out of town with a friend. Mary told me afterwards, "I did bring my air-spray out of habit, but my poop didn't really smell that bad."

Okay, then!

At the twenty-week follow-up when I asked her to estimate, Mary reported feeling sixty percent better.

She joyfully announced, "I'm going to Europe for the first time ever, Doctor! I'm 58, and I've never traveled overseas because of my poop problems! I am starting to smell freedom," she joked.

Symptoms of a Bloated Stomach

Bloating is different than gaining abdominal fat mass. It is often caused by trapped abdominal air and is usually temporary. It might feel like you have built-up gas in your digestive system, like your belly is "sticking out," or you may be in plain old *pain*. Other symptoms may include:

- Skin rashes or hives
- Vomiting or nausea

- Watery eyes, itchy throat, and other signs of an allergic reaction
- Constipation or diarrhea
- Blood in your urine or stool
- Unintentional weight loss
- Lymph node pain: including groin, throat or armpits
- Ongoing fatigue
- Brain fog and difficulty concentrating
- Hemorrhoids
- Irregular periods

The Many, Many *Causes* of a Bloated Belly . . .

There are dozens, if not hundreds, of different (usually hidden) reasons for a bloated belly. These include bacteria imbalances (dysbiosis), overuse of antibiotics, allergies, hormonal imbalances, thyroid dysfunction, and more. It can be hard to pinpoint the main offender, but an excellent chronological history along with detailed information about one's reactions to different foods (and circumstances) will usually increase the chances of determining someone's bloating triggers.

Excessive gas is very common. And a bloated belly from regular bouts with excess gas usually indicates a problem with digestion, especially once other causes have been ruled out. Various factors can contribute to stomach bloating, including some that may seem unconnected, such as lack of sleep or excessive stress. Excessive gas in the intestines is often the result of:

- Improper protein digestion, leading some foods to ferment in the body
- Weakened ability to efficiently break down sugar and carbohydrates
- Imbalances in gut bacteria

With trillions of healthy and unhealthy bacteria competing for survival, sometimes the "bad bacteria" can outweigh the good, and *dysbiosis* (an imbalance of bacteria in the gut) occurs, leading to abdominal gas and discomfort.

Could It Have A Medical Reason?

Bloating may be due to any number of medical conditions. These include:

- Irritable bowel syndrome
- Inflammatory bowel diseases, such as ulcerative colitis or Crohn's disease
- Functional gastrointestinal disorders (FGIDs)
- Heartburn
- Food intolerance/sensitivity
- Weight gain
- Hormonal flux (especially for women)
- Intestinal parasite infections, such as Giardia
- Eating disorders: anorexia nervosa, bulimia nervosa or others
- Emotional factors: stress, anxiety, depression, and more
- Certain medications
- Fluid retention

CASE STUDY

Joanne: "I'm Even Passing Gas Through My Vagina!"

One of my patients, Joanne, presented with a classic case of bloating caused by fluid retention. She was a 47-year-old nurse with "a sweet tooth and an addiction to fast food."

She first came to my office when she noticed that her jewelry and clothes were becoming too tight. She was experiencing severe mood swings. She'd also developed swelling and pain around her joints, her face was puffy—and, she added with extreme embarrassment, "I'm even passing gas through my vagina."

Joanne had recently gone through a pregnancy that required an emergency C-section due to preeclampsia, a condition in pregnant women indicated by high blood pressure, sometimes with fluid retention and an increased, dangerous level of protein in the urine. In Joanne's case, she also presented with a high fever, leading her obstetric team to load her up with antibodies to protect her and the baby. Because of the high doses of the antibiotic, Joanne had developed an exceedingly unbalanced microbiome, a detail missed by her previous medical team.

After testing her microbiome and identifying the imbalance and the severe damage it had done to her system, I convinced Joanne to cut sugar and fast food from her diet.

The first step was to balance her neurohormones, which are chemical messenger molecules that are released in the blood system by neurons and are vital for development, growth, reproduction, feeding and behavior. Their imbalance likely contributed to Joanne's up-and-down moods. The second was to start treating Joanne with antifungals for her candida overgrowth by putting her on the Johns Hopkins protocol, which proved to be successful for her. On her six-month visit, Joanne walked in smiling. "I've finally gotten rid of those nasty little critters in my stomach! My body—my 'temple' as you asked me to look at it—is on the mend, and it's clearer than it has ever been."

Dehydration

One of the first questions I ask my patients when they tell me about their bloating symptoms is "How much water are you drinking daily?"

So often, people are not consuming even *close* to enough water to meet the daily requirement. Every day, a person should drink, in ounces, half of their body weight in pounds. For example, a 150 lb. person needs 75 ounces of water per day.

Not drinking enough water, eating a lot of salty foods, or drinking an excess of alcohol can lead to dehydration.[2] If you aren't drinking enough fluids, your body will actually retain water to prevent dehydration from occurring. So, in order to avoid this dehydration situation in the first place, DRINK MORE WATER!

Constipation

Now, this will go hand-in-hand with dehydration. Constipation occurs when our poop gets stuck in the intestines, which happens when you aren't drinking enough water or when you're not eating enough fiber-rich foods.[3] It can happen to the best of us. We try so hard to poop; we know we have to, but nothing comes out. In another chapter, I'll list the foods you can eat to prevent bloating and constipation in detail, including fiber-rich foods.

SIBO

SIBO occurs when bad bacteria invades and grows in the small intestine, wreaking havoc on our gut and causing our microbiome to become out of balance. The most common symptoms of SIBO are bloating and increased gas production. One common reason is the overuse of antibiotics.[4]

Hormonal Changes

I have devoted a whole chapter to this very important topic because it is vital to the successful treatment of bloating. Hormone imbalances, especially in women, can cause extreme symptoms. Most people know that PMS commonly causes fluid retention and bloating.[5] However, if the bloating that often follows a PMS flare does not go away after a few days, then perhaps the hormones are out of whack!

Other Serious Causes

Abdominal bloating can be a symptom of several other serious conditions, including:

- Pathologic fluid accumulation in the abdominal cavity, called *ascites*, due to certain cancers, liver disease, kidney failure, or congestive heart failure
- Celiac disease (gluten intolerance)
- Pancreatic insufficiency (which impairs digestion because the pancreas does not produce sufficient digestive enzymes)
- A perforated GI tract (leaking gas, normal GI bacteria, and other contents into the abdominal cavity)

Bloating and gas are *usually* tied to what—and how—you eat. Understanding why it is happening to your body, and then making changes to your diet and lifestyle can go a long way for most people. I do caution you. In some cases, bloating might be a sign of a more significant medical issue. That is why I recommend that people with bloating seek medical help from someone who understands the many possible causes of bloating.

A Word About Genomics

There has recently been an increased interest in the genetic makeup of the gut bacteria that cause bloating. The consensus is that the molecular makeup of bacteria can, when out of balance, contribute to bloating. The astounding diversity of the bacteria in our gut functions collectively, in a well-ordered environment, with each group of bacteria playing a specific and vital role for us as their hosts.

This area of study, called Genomics, involves the mapping of gut bacteria to characterize our individual genetics as well as the relationship between disease and a weakened microbiome.

The finding that particular bacteria with certain molecular structures are present in people with bloating suggests that specific molecular differences are passed down through the generations. For example, during natural childbirth when the baby passes through the birth canal, they may ingest the mother's bacteria. Research has proven that babies born vaginally have a different microbiome (gut bacteria) when compared to babies delivered by caesarean. Vaginally born babies get most of their gut bacteria from their mother via the vaginal canal, whereas babies born via cesarean have been shown to have bacteria associated with hospital environments in their guts. Although more research is needed to see if these different birth methods have any effect on later health, a significant body of research already says it does. For example, research states for example, that babies with disrupted microbiome secondary to a cesarean delivery, early antibiotic use, or no (or limited) breastfeeding are at greater risk for many medical conditions, including allergies, asthma, other respiratory infections, irritable bowel disease, SIBO, and even obesity and type 1 diabetes. However, parents still optimize a baby's bacterial ecosystem no matter how the birth took place.[6,7]

There Is Hope For All

People from all walks of life visit me in my office, from those who are newly experiencing bloating, to those who have dealt with horrible symptoms for the majority of their lives. I want you to know that there is hope for anyone and everyone—even someone who feels that bloating has taken over their whole life.

To fully understand why bloating affects us so deeply, it is imperative that we understand its relationship with bacteria—and the gut.

CASE STUDY

Julian: The Soiled-Pants Basketball Player

Julian was 64 years old, a new patient, and had been misdiagnosed with IBS (irritable bowel syndrome) 15 years ago. He described his first episode as being ". . .nothing short of horrible and devastating! I was at a pick-up basketball game. It just came on like a tornado, and I just didn't make it to the bathroom in time. Doc, I soiled my shorts in front of *all these dudes*! I've been kind of traumatized ever since."

Julian had never been given a definitive reason for his ongoing symptoms: swollen belly, excessive gas, and explosive diarrhea.

He went on to say, "I was so horrified that it would happen again that I quit the dream job I'd loved for twenty years because it required me to travel too much. I kept having nightmares before every trip about being on the plane and not making it to the restroom in time. I even tried wearing diapers on my flights, but I still had to live with the humiliating noise from passing gas."

Julian's anxiety played such a huge role in triggering his

episodes that his marriage eventually fell apart. "My two adult daughters are totally fed up with me because they think I'm overly-obsessed with my bathroom habits." He went on, "But I worry so much about having an accident that it causes me even *more* anxiety and makes an accident even more likely."

It's a confounding vicious circle! The more anxiety, the more the accident potential! Classic with this syndrome.

Julian's laboratory results showed that he had a slew of food sensitivities—some so severe that I was surprised he hadn't had an anaphylactic response. Also, due to his previous bout with alcohol abuse (and the insane amount of ibuprofen he had taken to help him with his hangovers), Julian's microbiome was shot. His bad bacteria had so overwhelmed his system that his inflammation was off the charts. He'd joined an online IBS support group, lamenting, "I found no one had symptoms as bad as I had, and the members were mostly women. I thought I was really f*@#ed up!"

He'd even tried avoiding trigger foods and beverages, but he'd occasionally fall off the wagon. And whatever small gains he'd made would go right down the drain. Unfortunately, antidiarrheal and anti-anxiety meds provided no relief whatsoever.

I was surprised that Julian had even come to me. I don't think I've ever seen someone who considered himself such a hopeless case. I started by assuring Julian that he was not "doomed for life," as he saw himself. With Julian's sports background in mind, I smiled and said, "Let's work as a team and, 'win this one for the Gipper.'"

This perked him up, so we talked about a program for him. We invited his live-in girlfriend, Connie, to join us after he told me, "She's my most reliable and most understanding support because she dealt with something similar a while ago."

We started Julian on the *Reset Cleanse Program* that I have created as part of my protocol for treatment. I put him on the herbs recommended in the Johns Hopkins' SIBO study (which will be described later in the book), as well as on an antifungal and antiparasitic medication. Parasites were the most likely reason for his poop "smelling like a dead animal," as he described it.

Once his SIBO breath test came in—one of the highest levels I had ever seen—we decided to give Julian a trial of rifaximin (an antibiotic that treats diarrhea, IBS, or other digestive issues) to provide him with a head start on the integrative protocol I had designed for him.

Acupuncture was the next step, followed by a DNA genetic test to evaluate him for possible DNA mutations, which occur as part of our evolution for the survival of our species. Sometimes these mutations can lead to "defects" in the sequence of our DNA, leading an array of medical conditions, some benign, some not. Julian's genetic test revealed that he had a mutation in the "methylation pathway," which is the body's main pathway to self-detox. In Julian's case, his Methylenetetrahydrofolate Reductase (MTHFR), the primary enzyme in the pathway, was only working ten percent of the time. This meant that his body was so overwhelmed with toxins and inflammation that everything would eventually fail, no matter what Julian did to counteract his symptoms. So, the next approach was to treat his MTHFR problem.

During his three-month follow-up, Julian reported that his symptoms had improved by only about fifteen percent, but it was enough for him to feel hopeful. "This is the first time in years that I see the 'light at the end of the tunnel!'"

Then, I started him on weekly IV drips of Glutathione, considered the most potent scavenger and antioxidant for the body. At month nine of his treatment, Julian and Connie booked a two-week vacation in Hawaii. He called me from his hotel and said in a discouraged voice, "The first few days were a dream, but then I got so excited about feeling so good that I decided to have a couple Pina Coladas and some sushi. My symptoms are back with a vengeance! I'm considering taking a red-eye home."

I was able to talk him off the ledge; I instructed Julian that, except for water, he should fast for 24 hours. He felt better. Julian jumped "back on the wagon" and avoided triggering foods, and his symptoms improved. Julian and Connie were able to enjoy the rest of their trip without further incident.

In addition to the nutritional changes, Julian incorporated stress management changes. He even tried breathing exercises and started meditating. Twelve months into his "total lifestyle makeover," as he loved to say, Julian reported that his symptoms were 75% better. He added, "Whatever the thing is that makes meditation so powerful, it's definitely working for me. I'm back playing golf with my buddies, which is precisely what I love to do."

Bacteria: Friend or Foe?

*"The ever-mysterious role of gut bacteria; it can optimize gut
health like no other, but it can also easily kill you."*

—E. de Mello, MD, PhD

The human condition is marked with many contradictions:
"Less is more." "Big is the new small." And bacteria are
no different. We seem simultaneously terrified by and obsessed
with them.

Even before we were thinking about Covid-19, many of us
avoided germs and bacteria. Then, we decided to spend billions of dollars annually on designer probiotics—which *grow*
bacteria—and ingest them, on purpose.

Global sales of probiotics rose more than 48%; from 2.7 billion dollars in 2011, to 4 billion dollars in 2016, with the strongest
growth occurring in the US.[1] In fact, the sales of probiotics by
2024 is projected to surpass 6 billion dollars.[2]

Still, some of us do everything we can to avoid unnecessary
encounters with the nasty little critters that can make our lives
miserable. We hate germs!

But the truth is, *we are like walking petri dishes.*

It's true. We humans are rife with bacterial colonies. From
our skin to the deepest recesses of our gut, we play host to
both "good" and "bad" bacteria. These bacteria perform complex and essential functions in our everyday lives. The "good"

bacteria have an essential function in keeping us healthy. In fact, without bacteria and other microorganisms, the world and the humans who inhabit it would likely cease to exist.

Bacteria is vital to our existence, as it performs critical functions on our behalf. It harvests nutrients and develops the immune system. Bacteria are actually *essential* for human survival on our planet.

But what else are they doing to me?

To accomplish their tasks and to survive, microbes in the gastrointestinal tract are also under pressure to manipulate their host's behavior—meaning *they try to fool your brain*! They want to make sure we feed them what *they* want. They do this by generating cravings and inducing anxiety until the individual in question eats what the bacteria wants and craves, whether or not the desired food is healthy for us! It might feel like we don't even have a choice. This is why many people with overeating behavior issues succumb to their microbiome's demands, despite their honest attempts to use willpower.

The truth is, it's not even a fair fight.

Microbes control the vagus nerve, which sends a Bluetooth-like signal back and forth between the gut and the brain. Evidence shows that they can have dramatic effects on our behavior. Microbes can even influence production of mood-altering toxins, as well as create changes in our taste receptors. These little critters exert quite a powerful influence on our reward and satiety pathways, so they can even have an effect on how much we want to eat. Evidence shows that microbes can have dramatic effects on behavior through this microbe driven gut-brain axis.[3]

Love Me, Love Me Not . . .

But why do we have a love-hate relationship with bacteria? (As if we needed any more complicated relationships in our lives!)

They love us because they *need us* in order to survive. Just like that old "ex" in some of our lives, bacteria and other microbes simply cannot leave us alone! Bacteria can fail to get the message that enough is enough, and then they turn against us—causing health issues for the very people feeding them.

Given the opportunity, bacteria will simply just take over. It becomes a war for the survival of the fittest. They can grow to the point that they "hijack" your system, acting like the host while we play guests in our own bodies! This love-hate relationship begins at birth.

As soon as we are born, many mothers will do everything in their power to keep those microscopic-sized little suckers away from their babies! But newborns ingest mouthfuls of bacteria, even during birth. Additionally, babies pick up plenty more from their mother's skin and milk during breastfeeding, when the mammary glands become colonized with bacteria. Our interaction with our mother is the most significant burst of microbes that we get in life.

Starting in the mouth, nose, or other orifices (guess which other orifices!), these microbes travel through the esophagus, stomach, and finally to the intestines where most of them set up camp.

Although there are estimated to be more than five hundred species of bacteria living in an adult intestine at any one time, the majority belong to two categories of living organisms: the *Firmicutes* (which include *Streptococcus Clostridium* and *Staphylococcus*), and the *Bacteroidetes* (which include *Flavobacterium*).[4,5]

Some researchers have argued that because some of our genes aren't found in our closest animal ancestors, they must have been transferred to humans from bacteria somewhat recently in our evolutionary history. So, even our genes are associated with bacteria. According to the Human Genome Project, published in 2001, about forty human genes evolved from bacteria.[6]

Bad Gut, Bad Mood?

The idea that the brain and the gut are so interconnected is not a surprise. Think of popular phrases in our everyday language: "gut instincts" for when we're experiencing intuition, or if we're brave, we are called "gutsy." In other words, we attribute several human emotions directly to our gut.

There have been a handful of studies exploring whether or not the effect of bacteria in the gut-brain axis may be scientifically observed in humans. For a recent double-blind study published in the journal, *Brain, Behavior, and Immunity*, researchers at Leiden University in the Netherlands recruited forty healthy volunteers.[7] The study was funded by a probiotic manufacturer. For one month, twenty of the volunteers took a probiotic containing a mix of eight strains of bacteria. The other half of the volunteers were given a placebo that looked exactly the same.

To assess the probiotic's effect on vulnerability to "sad" moods, each of the participants filled out questionnaires at both the beginning and the end of the study. They were asked to rate how strongly they agreed with statements like "When I'm in a sad mood, I think about how my life could be different," or "When I'm down, I more often feel overwhelmed by things."

The head researcher of the study and her colleagues found that those in the group taking the probiotic tended to answer these questions very differently at the end of the study than they had at the beginning. They reported experiencing less aggressive and ruminative thoughts, and they were less reactive to their own negative thoughts and feelings.

This study shows that probiotics may be influential in positively affecting moods for those who are vulnerable to sadness—which provides further evidence for the existence of the gut-brain connection. Clearly, we must pay more attention. Our gut is influential in more ways than we previously thought!

3

The Amazing Gut: A Beehive-like System

*"Good bacteria is to good digestion what good
pollination is to delicious honey."*

—E. de Mello, MD, PhD

Have you ever seen a beehive? What does a beehive need to
maximize its growth and production of honey? The more
healthy bees in a hive, the more opportunity there is for pollen gathering and, therefore, honey production. The hive is the
bees' home. To proliferate and provide us with the tasty honey
we love, bees need shelter and safety. A good beekeeper provides
an environment that meets or exceeds the needs they seek out
in nature.

A Bee's Needs:
- Bees need food in the form of pollen on flowers.
- Bees need the ability to expand their numbers.
- Bees need dry and well-ventilated conditions.
- Bees need a nearby source of water.

In essence, bees need precisely what our microbiome needs:
food, the ability to reproduce, good growth conditions, and
water.

What is a Microbiome, and Why Does it Exist?

Within the complex physiological, biochemical and hormonal interactions that define us as humans, the organ that most integrates our body with the outside world is the digestive system. In short, the gut.

The gut is the foundation of our immune system. The gut is continuously exposed to new microbes and molecules that come from the things we eat and drink, and it is heavily influenced by our outside environment, including the city we live in, how much stress we put on ourselves, as well as diet and exercise.[1]

The gut plays a vital function in the central nervous system and brain, and as discussed, it even influences your mood!

"How can it do that?" you might ask. Well, because of the interactions between ourselves and the trillions of bacteria that make up the microbiome.[2]

Because of the sensitivity of our microbiome environment and how easily its contents can be affected, it is imperative we practice care and caution with our gut and understand exactly what we put into our bodies and what we're exposing our bodies to.

How Do Healthy Bacteria in the Microbiome Benefit Our Health?

The notion of good bacteria being essential to good health has reemerged in the last two decades, with an increasing body of research showing that beneficial microorganisms play a crucial role in how well our bodies and brains function. The numerous bacteria in our digestive tract have an "operating agreement" with us. In exchange for us feeding them, they support the breakdown and metabolism of nutrients, vitamin absorption, and waste processing, in exchange for us feeding them. The evidence that the mix of bacteria populating the gut influences our susceptibility and immunity to disease is now well documented. This is true for physical conditions such as asthma and emotional health.

The Bacteria Milky Way

Current research suggests our gut contains anywhere between forty and one hundred trillion bacteria. How does one comprehend the vastness of such a number? This is hundreds of times more than even the number of stars in our Milky Way Galaxy. There are more bacterial organisms in our bodies than there are stars in the sky. In that sense, human beings can be considered more bacterial than skin and bones. When we take a giant step into the microscopic realm, our body is the home to a virtual "bacterial universe."[3,4,5,6]

Another remarkable revelation of how essential bacteria is to our health has recently been discovered. A study from the University of Calgary's Cumming School of Medicine, published in the journal, *Cell*, reveals a new mechanism in how the gut microbiome regulates anti-inflammatory cells. A protein expressed in bacteria called *Bacteroides* works to prevent IBD by rapidly recruiting white blood cells to kill a rogue part of the immune system that is responsible for causing IBD.[7]

Furthermore, a significant body of research has attested to the critical role of bacteria in the communication of the gut-brain axis, proposing that certain organisms may aid in the treatment of stress-related disorders such as anxiety and depression. One is the vagus nerve—which extends from the GI tract to the brain, sending signals back and forth between these intrinsically connected organs.[8]

The Importance of the Microbiome

The microbiome is so central to how the body functions, some scientists treat it as its own organ system. The microbiome has widespread impact on aging, digestion, the immune system, mood, and cognitive function in the body.

In fact, the study of the microbiome dates back centuries. Antonie van Leewenheck, a Dutch scientist, studied his own oral and fecal microbiota in the 1680s and observed just how different the environments of each were.[9] Through other observations, he saw that healthy and diseased microbiota were different from each other. Because we have this information, we can further investigate just how diseases change our microbiomes from a healthy state to a diseased one.[10]

As our bodies grow and mature, our microbiomes learn with age how to deal with certain types of bacteria. Upon years of exposure to bacteria, our microbiome will determine whether microbes that enter our body are harmful or beneficial and deal with them accordingly.[11] Our bodies have been exposed to bacteria since birth. If born vaginally, we will be exposed to the *Lactobacillus* bacteria; if born by Caesarean section, we are exposed to *Staphylococcus*, *Corynebacterium*, and *Propionibacterium*, which are skin bacteria.[12] After birth, the amount of bacteria we harbor in our microbiome will exponentially increase. As newborns, we only have about 100 species of microbes, but by the time we get to age 3, we harbor more like 1000 species.[13] As we grow into adulthood, the number of species only increases.

The Microbiome-Brain Connection and Bloating

Bacteria is about the survival of the fittest. As I mentioned earlier, they can nudge you to eat what they need to survive—a high-carbohydrate diet that can lead to insulin resistance, bloating, and SIBO. When this happens, blood sugar surges, leading to the depletion of neurotransmitters, essential B vitamins, and magnesium. This depletion causes stress on the liver, further worsening the body's ability to detox while increasing food sensitivities and bloating.

4

Candida Overgrowth: Microbiome Gone Wrong

"Candida overgrowth is not an illness. Rather it is a condition caused by an imbalance of our microbiome."
—E. de Mello, MD, PhD

What the Heck is Candida?

Candida is a type of yeast; a single-celled microorganism that *loves* humans because without us, this annoying bug could not live. Candida is opportunistic because it overgrows at every opportunity—especially when the host is immunocompromised.

It grows when we "feed it," like savoring too many sugary desserts. It loves to overgrow (like weeds) in our mouths, intestinal tracts, on our skin and—*Yikes!*—in the genital area, where it can be passed from person to person during sex.

Symptoms of Candida Overgrowth

Candida is classified as fungi. This phylum (or category) also includes mushrooms, mold, and mildew. In balanced amounts, fungi are part of our microbiome, our normal flora. We all have Candida in our gut. But Candida is very selfish in that it takes all it can but does not give us anything back. It doesn't support or improve our overall health and well-being at all. Instead,

THE CANDIDA GROWTH CYCLE

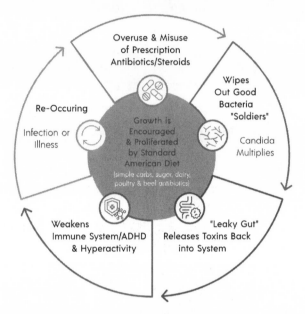

when it becomes overgrown, it causes significant symptoms to flare up.

The symptoms of Candida overgrowth include bloating, constipation, diarrhea, abdominal pain and cramping, increased gas production, recurring vaginal yeast infections, chronic UTIs (urinary tract infections), chronic fatigue syndrome, and the ever hard-to-resist sugar and carbohydrate cravings! The symptoms can range anywhere from mild to severe, and they vary from person to person.

Generally, unless the human host has a compromised immune system, as with cancer or HIV, a Candida infection isn't life-threatening, but it can make us feel horrible all the same. Joint pain, muscle aches, anxiety and depression, mood swings, irritability, recurring sinus infections, difficult-to-pinpoint chronic inflammation, brain fog, and restless sleep are also common symptoms. If Candida is left untreated, it can spread to the bloodstream causing *Invasive Candidiasis*, a serious infection that can affect the blood, vital organs, and even your bones.

Candida overgrowth can also lead to an excess of other opportunistic microbes in the gut, so it might be hard to tell which sneaky culprit is causing the most harm. No wonder bloating can be so hard to diagnose!

Main Causes of Candida

1. A Compromised Immune System

In my clinical practice, I have found that Candida overgrowth occurs when there is a disruption in the immune system. A sugary or carbohydrate-based diet, processed foods, environmental toxicity, lack of sleep, dehydration, and stress all impair the immune system and create the perfect environment for Candida microbes to take over your system. This compromises your "good bugs" (good flora), thus allowing the bad bacteria to dominate.

CANDIDA OVERGROWTH STAGES

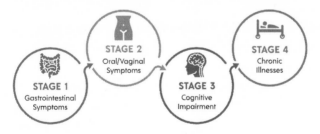

STAGE 1
Gastrointestinal
Symptoms

STAGE 2
Oral/Vaginal
Symptoms

STAGE 3
Cognitive
Impairment

STAGE 4
Chronic
Illnesses

2. Overuse of Antibiotics

This is a scary problem that's affecting the whole world. Few people realize that antibiotics have become one of our biggest threats. The overuse of antibiotics in humans and other animals is rapidly destroying our ability to defend ourselves against disease. According to the World Health Organization, antibiotic resistance now threatens not only the global health of the world's population, but the health of the planet itself. Economically speaking, antibiotic resistance leads to longer hospital stays, higher medical costs, and increased mortality.[1]

We now know, for sure, that the overuse of antibiotics kills beneficial bacterial species in the gut. When this happens, the balance of microbes that help our system weakens, creating the perfect condition for Candida overgrowth.[2]

3. Dysbiosis (Gut Dysfunction)

There are many scientific studies that link leaky gut syndrome, IBS (irritable bowel system), IBD, and SIBO—all of which cause bloating—to Candida overgrowth. In fact, leaky gut, bloating, and Candida often occur concurrently. Candida releases toxins that trigger inflammation throughout the body. This inflammation can damage the gut lining, exacerbate leaky gut, and cause bloating.

4. Our "Carb-Crazy," Overloaded Diet

Looking at the high incidence of obesity, diabetes, and heart disease in the Western World (with the United States leading the pack), it's evident that the ever-growing problem of Candida can be partially blamed on our poor diets. Neither natural nor nourishing to our bodies, refined sugar and carbohydrates act as high-octane fuel sources for Candida and lead to rapid overgrowth. When you feed these goodies to Candida, you are giving Candida the little snacks it needs to grow, while simultaneously promoting the microbiome disruption that robs your immune system of its effectiveness to counter the problem. In other words, when we encourage Candida to grow by feeding it its favorite foods, we impair our immune system's ability to maintain a healthy symbiotic relationship with Candida, not to mention the numerous other aggressive microbes we might have to battle.

5. Environmental Toxins

Another major cause of Candida overgrowth is exposure to environmental and chemical toxins. This exposure to an ever-growing number of chemicals in homes, schools, at work, and in the general environment can lead to hormonal imbalances and, eventually, immunosuppression.

I find it especially scary to read almost daily about food recalls, oil spills, and the dumping of chemical waste into our water, causing severe disruptions in our ecosystem.

In addition, mold, found in many homes, is another type of yeast and is a close relative of Candida. Mycotoxins, or mold spores and mold metabolites, can also be present in the air, especially under very moist conditions. When inhaled, these spores can suppress your immune system and encourage Candida overgrowth, which can produce its *own* mycotoxins that can make you feel terribly sick.

A Short List of Common Toxins:

- **Phthalates:** endocrine-disrupting chemicals used to make plastics flexible
- **Biphenyl A:** another endocrine disruptor found in food and drink containers, can linings, and store receipts
- **Radon:** an odorless, radioactive gas that can seep into homes from the ground
- **PFCs (Perfluorochemicals):** used on stain-resistant fabrics (like Scotchgard®, Gore-tex®), cooking pans (Teflon®), food wrappers, and microwave popcorn bags
- **Flame retardants:** used in building materials, cushions, and more
- **Formaldehyde:** often found in building materials and pressed-wood furniture products
- **Lead:** found in a lot of paint made prior to 1978 and in old plumbing

- **Parabens:** estrogen imitators used in cosmetics and other beauty products
- **Chlorine:** a disinfectant commonly used in municipal water systems and swimming pools

Biofilm

A thin, slimy film of bacteria that adheres to a surface, biofilm is the microscopic sticky substance in which bacteria replicate and thrive. It clings to surfaces that we touch every day—like water bottles, counter tops, car and airplanes seats, kitchen tile—and yes, sometimes even doctors' dirty white coats!

As I already mentioned, it's true that we humans have a love-hate relationship with bacteria. We do everything we can to get rid of it, and then we go out and buy probiotic-infused drinks and take probiotic tablets to replace the good parts of the bacteria we have erased!

Aside from external biofilms, with which we often come into contact while living in toxic, over-populated settings, we also develop internal biofilms in our own GI tracts.

Although there are many types of both good and bad biofilm, in this chapter, I'll address only the kind that hosts non-beneficial bacteria in our system.

We ALL Have It

Humans normally have a safe amount of biofilm in their bodies—not enough to cause any medical conditions unless the microbiome is out of balance. In the case of bloating due to SIBO or any other chronic GI condition, the microfilm becomes disproportionate. For total healing to occur, bacterial biofilm MUST be controlled.

There is always a certain amount of external biofilm in your work and home environment. This is why I use a probiotic cleaning product to clean my body, office, and home. The best way to rid the body of biofilm is to create a healthy environment by killing off non-beneficial bacteria and yeast while repopulating beneficial bacteria.

Dietary changes aimed at lowering sugar and carbohydrates are essential. Adding digestive enzymes, prebiotics and probiotics, and natural antimicrobials such as garlic to your regime (unless you are allergic), together with lifestyle modifications, will strengthen your immune system and sufficiently decrease bacterial biofilm.

How does biofilm contribute to bloating?

Although you may have just learned about it, you have likely come in contact with biofilm in a variety of ways. For example, on your teeth. The plaque that dental hygienists remove to avoid decay is an example of bacterial biofilm. The slimy stuff responsible for clogging the drains in your house is another example. So is the gooey film that causes rocks in a stream of water to be slippery. Biofilm is associated with a significant percentage of all infections, including the ones that cause bloating.

Sites for biofilm formation include many kinds of surfaces, such as metals, plastics, and medical implant materials. You may not be surprised that bacteria biofilms are also found in the nasal passageways.

Given that the GI tract has an ongoing availability of nutrients that bacteria need to thrive, bacteria, fungi, and associated biofilms like to attach to it. The walls of our gut (gut epithelium) are lined with mucus for self-protection. In patients with ongoing inflammation, including bloating, this self-protective mechanism is disrupted, causing the bacteria to attach directly to the gut wall and form biofilm.[3]

But, as I said, not all biofilms are harmful. They play crucially beneficial roles in ecosystems by decomposing and recycling organic material. This keeps nutrients circulating in the marine food chain in our oceans, thereby creating a vital metabolic cooperability. The key is balance.

5

Nutrition

"Diseases run in families because
EATING HABITS run in families."

—Unknown

Nearly every week, a new study or new claims about diet and health make headlines. Opinions about nutrition are as abundant as they are confusing. Keeping up with what will help us live to be one hundred and what will kill us can be daunting.

"Is Sugar Toxic?" screamed the New York Times in 2011, and *"Eat Butter!"*—an equally blunt statement—appeared on the cover of Time Magazine in 2014. With astounding regularity, we hear about a previously "good" food or supplement that, for one reason or another, suddenly becomes an evil food.

Take the egg. Through the eighties, it was considered the perfect breakfast. During the nineties it was declared pure poison. But, today, it has been re-blessed and is back on most recommended lists again. But an egg is still an egg. It didn't change its molecular structure back and forth over the years. So, what is happening?

It's frustrating to be a consumer. We wonder, "What the heck am I supposed to eat? Or not eat? Who's telling the truth? And who is just trying to sell me something?"

Food and Gas: What's the Connection?

While certain foods allow different good bacteria to thrive, others impact us negatively. We have all experienced that certain foods can make us gassy. Many of us have also experienced a sudden episode of bloating when we change what we eat too quickly. The reason is that the microbiota, the trillions of bacteria in the gut, usually need time to adjust to a new diet. But that is not necessarily true for all people.

More sensitive people may have a rapid change in the populations of their microbiota when they change their diets, while some people can maintain diversity with more stability. I often hear patients complain about gas after experimenting with foods that they don't usually eat. This happens a lot when we travel and surprise our bodies with an exotic meal. Or it can even happen when we eat an unusually fiber-heavy meal.

Bacteria in our gut naturally create gas as they ferment what we eat to more efficiently digest our food. That's why the average person passes gas at least fourteen times a day.

What the Hell DO I Eat?

"One man's food is someone else's poison."
—James L. D'Adamo

Everyone is biologically different, although as humans, our basic nutritional requirements are somewhat similar. How we process those nutrients required by our system varies from person to person.

A perfect example of this is the common peanut. A source of protein for some people—a death-knell for others, if they are allergic. And, excuse me Generation Z, but when we were children, we were instructed to "drink three glasses of milk every day" to fulfill our daily calcium requirements. Hah!

Nowadays, it seems half the population is "lactose intolerant." And milk isn't the only culprit. All dairy products, including cheese, yogurt, etc., are an issue. The list goes on and on as to what some people cannot safely eat or drink.

As such, "the perfect diet" does not really exist, and the idea that there is a universal, perfect diet only adds confusion to a field already saturated with misinformation

How Do I Know What's Good for Me?

What a funny question actually. Animals in nature do not question what they eat. They just do it based on instinct. How is it that we have gotten so far removed from our true nature that we are lost and clueless about what is good for us and what is not?

If you have trouble knowing what you should be eating, I recommend that you set up an appointment and talk to a nutritionist. After a comprehensive interview reviewing your family history, allergies, etc., a nutritionist will be able to design a *food program* to meet your needs—notice I didn't say that scary word, *"diet"*! Your program will be tailored precisely to fit you, and if followed, will likely lend to your experience of optimum health.

So many people try to follow the latest diet craze they read about on the internet, be it Paleo, Keto, Mediterranean, Atkins, Fruitarian, South Beach, Nutrisystem, Volumetrics, Macrobiotic, Master Cleanse, Scarsdale, Zone, or whatever. When a diet is not specifically designed for them (for example, by a nutritionist following a consultation) and they find that it does not work, they're likely to blame themselves, throw their arms up in the air, and say, "Forget this diet crap! I am going to eat whatever the heck I want." And then we are back to square one.

Common Sense About Eating
- **No matter what you're eating, do not eat too fast or too much.** We tend to *overeat* when we *eat too quickly*. This

is because there's a twenty-minute gap between satiation and fullness to the max. Think of Thanksgiving, when we wait for hours for that delicious, extravagant meal, and by the time we eat, we are so hungry that we eat non-stop, fast. Then we lay down and literally pass out. In other words, there is not time for the gut to acknowledge the important signs of fullness that tell you to stop eating *NOW*; you're full!

- **You are not chewing enough.** Chewing is important! Chewing adds salivary enzymes to food, which is a part of the digestion process. Chewing stimulates the stomach to produce more acid to help break down the food. Longer chewing, together with slower swallowing, leads to better digestion. According to studies on nutrition, it is best to chew each mouthful at least thirty times. I know how hard this is given our "on the go life." However, I guarantee that you will see a difference in your digestion and elimination if you were to commit to chew your food for at least half of the recommended time and swallow it slower. When you train yourself to eat more slowly, you automatically tend to chew your food more.

- **Eat high fiber foods** such as whole grains, bread, and oats. Fiber is good, right? This is a tricky one, as these may add to bloating, especially if you do not usually eat very much fiber.

- **Trapped air.** Chewing gum or drinking carbonated beverages causes us to consume air, which leads to bloating.

- **Lactose intolerance.** Lactase deficiency (not having enough of the enzyme responsible for digesting lactose) leads to nausea and/or bloating as soon as thirty minutes or up to two or three hours after consuming dairy products.

- **Gluten intolerance.** Individuals with celiac disease or who have gluten intolerance may experience bloating after eating foods with gluten-based products.

A Side Note on Excessive Gas

Yes, friends, gas is very common and is actually a sign that your gastrointestinal system is simply doing its job. In fact, when patients have major surgery, doctors do not usually let them move from the ICU or go home until they have passed gas. So, you shouldn't be at all surprised if your doctor comes to your bedside and asks, "Have you passed gas yet?" They are not being nosey or kinky—they're just making sure that your system is in working order. Passing gas is natural and nothing to be ashamed of. Everybody does it, and on average, 14 times a day![1]

Why can't I always smell it? As discussed, some gas comes from the air you swallow, through carbonated drinks, chewing gum, or eating too fast. So why are you not clearing the elevator when you let it out? Because the gas you pass is made mostly of the same odorless gas in the air: hydrogen.

When Does Passing Too Much Gas Become a Sign That Something is Wrong?

Once bacteria consume undigested and fermentable particles in the lower intestines, they cause overdrive fermentation.[2] But not all bacteria cause fermentation the same way. Some create more potent gas-makers than others, breaking down certain complex carbohydrates and sugars with odiferous results.

For example, bacteria that come from *sulfur-containing gases* (like hydrogen sulfide, methanethiol, and dimethyl sulfide) are common triggers of bloating and gas. However, while these pungent gases make up very little of the volume of a typical fart, your nose is extremely sensitive, and hence, you want to get out of that elevator at all costs when someone "cuts the cheese."[3]

The Vietnam Revenge

Thirty-two-year-old Yvonne had no significant medical health issues until recently. But this day, she walked into my office, sat down, apologized for being beside herself, and started sobbing.

"I am lost, doctor. My life has been miserable. Things basically revolve around never being too far from a bathroom. I pass gas all the time, very loudly. I go from constipation to diarrhea in a matter of two days. I'm so embarrassed! And I belch like a sea lion. I can't go on like this!"

I handed Yvonne a tissue. She dried her eyes and continued. "I was having the time of my life! Living a full, productive life, and dating. That was until about six months ago, when I went on a trip to Vietnam with my boyfriend, who has since broken up with me. He said it was because I'd become so moody and depressed."

The tears began to flow again. "I think the truth was that he couldn't handle my farting all the time! You know, dudes are expected to fart. They even have contests where they fart on demand. But women? God forbid if we fart! It is so not sexy. We're seen as slobs, not ladylike. I hate this double standard. But although I hate to admit it, I can't really blame him. Who wants to have sex with a woman who makes loud, pungent farts all the time?"

I inquired about her Vietnam trip. Yvonne said, "While we were over there, I decided to try some new foods. I even ate snake, which is considered a delicacy in some villages. Also, I started drinking milk again because my boyfriend convinced me that raw milk is the best."

"How did that affect you?" I asked.

"Not so good. I used to be a fairly strict vegetarian," she

said, "but almost immediately after eating snake meat and drinking raw milk, I started bloating like crazy." She indicated her distended stomach, then added, "I had several episodes of diarrhea, alternating with constipation, and my skin broke out with hives and acne."

She looked down at her stomach again lamenting, "I still feel like a miserable pregnant lady." Yvonne let out a deep sigh. "It got so bad that I decided to come home early, while my boyfriend stayed on without me. We'd planned on traveling Southeast Asia for three months. I left after less than thirty days."

Yvonne's stool test revealed that her digestive enzymes were, in fact, deficient, and her microbiome entirely out of balance with an overgrowth of yeast (Candida) and parasites. Her SIBO breath test was also off the charts.

The first step of the treatment involved giving her GI system a break. It was recommended that she not eat any uncooked high-fiber foods and drink only room temperature water with a few drops of lemon. She had to eliminate all sugars, including fruits (except for blackberries and blueberries), and no red meat, dairy products, or wheat. She was instructed to gradually start intermittent fasting as described in the Reset Program, first for four hours, then six, then eight hours.

I also had her place a hot water bottle on her belly every night. She did this for twenty minutes with a ten-minute break, repeating the cycle for a total of two hours to keep her belly warm and unrestricted. She was to "keep the fire in the belly," as practitioners of Chinese Medicine often recommend in order to increase blood flow to the gut. I also encouraged Yvonne to resume her exercise and yoga, but not to do sit-ups or put any pressure on her belly.

A month later, Yvonne reported feeling somewhat better. Her bloating and flatus had improved, and she was no longer constipated, although the diarrhea persisted. I started her on an herbal protocol for SIBO and a low FODMAP diet. (I will elaborate more on this later.)

On her sixty-day follow-up, Yvonne walked in and smiled broadly. "I am slowly getting my life back." She said her symptoms had decreased by fifty percent. Her diarrhea was less frequent, and her skin was recovering from "This f@#ing assault," as she put it.

I encouraged her to stay on the same regimen for another thirty days. Yvonne came back eight weeks later, beaming. "I am back in action, Doc!"

What's a FODMAP, and Why do I Care?

FODMAP: *Fermentable Oligosaccharides, Disaccharides, Monosaccharides, and Polyols.*

Whew! That's a mouthful. (Kinda makes you glad there's an acronym for it!) These are short-chain carbohydrates and sugar alcohols that are poorly absorbed by the body, frequently resulting in abdominal pain and bloating.

FODMAPs can be present in foods naturally or as additives. Examples of FODMAP food include beans, wheat and other grains, fructose, dairy, some legumes, and others.

FODMAPs are known for being difficult to digest. Many carbohydrates fall into this category. For many people, these types of carbohydrates are poorly tolerated, as they resist breakdown in the upper GI tract, feeding the bad bacteria in our lower gut. Lactose, fructose, and sugar alcohols are prime examples of FODMAPs, as are raffinose and stachyose—the byproducts of beans—that have a reputation for clearing the elevator after we consume them. They don't bother everyone, but eating them can make some people fart nonstop!

Remember the old sayings . . . *"Whoever smelt it, dealt it,"* and *"Whoever said the rhyme, did the crime!"*

Whether we are looking around for someone else to blame or not, reducing FODMAP consumption has scientifically been shown to diminish bloating and flatulence in individuals who are more susceptible to excessive or painful gas caused by fermentable foods.[4]

A low FODMAP diet is also known to relieve GI symptoms in individuals suffering with SIBO, IBS, Leaky Gut Syndrome, Crohn's disease, celiac disease and other gastrointestinal maladies.

Well-Known Gas-Producing Foods

I once read a funny article on foods that lead to "ass gas." It described them as so famous that they should be in the Fart Food Hall of Fame. With that in mind, let's look at some of the top gas-causing foods:

Dairy

Intestinal gas and bloating have been a common indicator of lactose intolerance and malabsorption for centuries. Surprise, surprise! Did you know that we are the only animals who drink milk after infancy? And to make it worse, we drink the milk of another species.

Who says we are meant to drink milk?

If you've answered, "the dairy industry," you win!

A person must have sufficient levels of enzymes in order to break down the sugars present in dairy products. This allows absorption into the bloodstream and their conversion into energy. If you don't have enough of these enzymes, eating lactose-ridden foods (milk, yogurt, ice cream, butter, cheese and dairy products, in general) will increase the not-so-friendly bacteria in your colon, and they will have a party there at your expense. And

after they feast, they leave the party room (your colon) a mess—
nasty, self-centered, little creeps that they are!

In other words, the lactose and proteins in dairy can worsen
digestive problems by feeding bad bacteria and triggering
inflammation in the lining of your gut.

Fructans

Fructans can be found in wheat, garlic, chickpeas, agave, artichokes, asparagus, leeks, shallots, onions, barley, broccoli,
jicama, and other foods. Foods, herbs, and spices that are high in
fructans are likely to cause painful digestive symptoms in those
who are fructan intolerant.

Garlic and Onions

Besides containing fructans, garlic and onion are high in sulfur,
which leads to those big stink-bombs. Choose low-FODMAP
herbs and spices such as *basil, cilantro, cumin, parsley, rosemary,
thyme, and turmeric* to flavor your food. The *green parts of scallions*
or green onions have also proven to be a safe option.

Beans and Legumes

Did you know that, botanically speaking, beans are considered a
legume? But beans are also a type of *seed*. And this seed—though
we don't usually call it this—is a type of *fruit*. To be ultra-specific,
beans are a type of legume that happens to be both a seed and a
fruit. To make it even more complex, beans can be consumed as
both a *vegetable* and *a protein*. What we know for sure about beans
is that they are famous worldwide for causing gas.

As previously mentioned, beans cause bloating (and subse-
quent farting) due to the high concentration of the FODMAP
carbs: alpha-gal (alpha galactose; in products made from mam-
mals), raffinose, and stachyose: all non-digestible, short-chain
carbohydrates.

Once a helping of beans lands in the gut, bacteria rapidly

break it down into the three main gases: CO_2, hydrogen, and methane. Although these gases are odorless, bacteria use the same sugars to make sulfur. And when they do, God save us . . . run for the exits! For certain people, the foul smell can be very intense and can last (and blast) for hours.

Wheat

How and why did our diet become so overloaded with wheat?

Given that approximately one percent of all Americans test positive for celiac disease, why is wheat so prevalent in the American diet? The answer: Money. That, and the fact that our taste buds have been manipulated by the food industry to crave more of what they are selling.

Studies have estimated that about twelve percent of people who do *not* test positive for celiac disease still report symptoms of digestive distress after eating foods with gluten. Add to this a 2018 study proposing that it is *not* actually gluten itself that causes the overwhelming array of issues in so many folks, but actually the fructans.[5]

The whole "gluten-is-bad-for-you" issue is extremely frustrating and confusing for a lot of people. While on one hand, certain healthcare professionals have loudly stated that gluten is "poison" and, hence, horrible for maintaining good health, on the other hand, others keep pounding us with the message that "whole wheat is essential for a daily balanced diet."

What is the truth?

The truth is, humans have been consuming wheat for thousands of years. How did an ancient food become junk food? Is it that modern wheat is worse than the wheat that granny ate? Since the beginning of civilization, this grain has been a staple in our diets. Easily cultivated and able to be stored for years in kernel form, this nutritional grain has been grown, harvested, and ground to make breads, pastas, and porridges all over the world.

But this ancient grain is not to blame for the array of medi-cal problems it causes. Rather, the problem is that today's wheat is vastly different from its original ancestors and even from the grain grown as recently as fifty or sixty years ago.

Wheat has changed through the industrialization of its plant-ing, growth, and storage. It is overly processed, its nutritional properties either erased or vastly diminished, and its stem has been made short (semi-dwarf wheat) for faster maturity, higher yield, and greater profit. In the old days, ancient wheat like Emmer, Einkorn and Khorasan (now known as Kamut) were the main variety of wheat consumed. Nowadays, almost *all* of the wheat commercially available is high-yield dwarf wheat. It was developed by crossbreeding and crude genetic manipulation in the 1960s.

How grains are processed first changed radically in the 1870s with the invention of the steel roller, which transformed grain milling forever. In 1879, at the beginning of the Industrial Revolution, the first steam mill was erected in London. The goal of this new method was to make grain milling fast, efficient, and cheaper. The finest form of flour could now be produced at a much lower cost.

This new process allowed every social class to enjoy what was to become known as "fancy flour." The new wheat and its derived "white flour" were celebrated as the new stars of modern cuisine everywhere. This new flour could be stored for a long time, and it traveled easily. Soon, wheat was everywhere. Wheat flour distribution chains sprouted all over the place, and the first processed foods were born. Vast numbers of shelf-stable foods were quickly produced in factories and readily transported to cities across the globe.

And the bugs won't eat it!

At first, it seemed like a good thing. Pesky insects rejected this new flour. What they did not realize back then was that this magical, modern milling method was destroying beneficial portions of the bran or wheat germ. The parts of the grain that were being destroyed (and still are) are rich in protein, lipids, minerals, and vitamins—the stuff we all need.

That's the reason why this new form of wheat flour was immune to pests! Stripped of its vital nutrients, even pesky bugs said, "No way am I eating that crap!" They knew better, before even we did!

Advancements in food production and farming in the twentieth century further cemented the damage being done to the ancient grain. In fact, the reduction of nutrient density in wheat coincides with the beginning of an increase in diseases that are known to be caused by spikes in blood sugar.

Stripped of what is called the "endosperm," where most of its nutritional elements are stored, wheat loses its value in the human diet. Separation of the bran and germ is the problem. Some are more sensitive than others, but people consuming processed wheat can eventually develop bothersome health issues, largely because many modern wheat products tend to spike sugar levels.

Sadly, even with the documented knowledge that wheat can become more unhealthy when it is stripped of its vital nutrients, this inferior, less expensive form remains highly popular in cuisines all over the world. All because today's industrialized wheat brings in billions of dollars annually, while also being cheaper for consumers.

High-Fructose Fruits

Fructose malabsorption, formerly known as *dietary fructose intolerance*, occurs when intestinal cells are unable to break down fructose efficiently. Fructose (the sugar found in fruit) is usually absorbed in the small intestine. Classified as a simple sugar and scientifically known as a *monosaccharide*, fructose is found mostly in fruit and some vegetables, but it is also found in honey, agave nectar, and in processed foods that contain added sugars.

In individuals with fructose intolerance, some amount of the sugar travels to the colon, where it is fermented by bacteria. The bloating, farting, and diarrhea that ensue are caused by the release of hydrogen and methane gases.

Research indicates that our fructose consumption (mostly from high fructose corn syrup) increased more than 1,000% between 1970 and 1990. This has contributed not only to the prevalent obesity in our culture, but also to an increase in fructose malabsorption and intolerance.

Fruits such as apples, cherries, mango, and watermelon are known to contain high levels of fructose sugars—as are sweeteners like coconut sugar and fruit juices. The problem is that not only can fructose feed your body's production of methane and hydrogen, but too much fructose can also compromise your liver function and is a shortcut to type 2 diabetes.

So, can I eat fruit?

Fruits are generally good nutrition, but they should be avoided when dealing with an unknown cause of bloating, except for low-fructose fruits, such as blueberries, blackberries, raspberries and strawberries.

Cruciferous Vegetables

These are high-sulfur vegetables that include broccoli, brussels sprouts, cabbage, bok choy, and cauliflower, which can be extremely gassy (and are common culprits of bloating) because they are packed with both fiber and raffinose. Cruciferous vegetables can cause high gas production and painful bloating and farting. In addition, these veggies also contain sulforaphane, which is broken down into the sulfurous compounds behind foul-smelling farts.[6]

Interestingly enough, this same sulforaphane can also help us prevent cancer, as it has recently been shown to selectively target and kill cancer cells. (Who could imagine that the same thing that causes smelly farts might one day prevent cancer?)[7] Cooking, fermenting, or steaming these particular veggies has been shown to break down their fiber, allowing for easier digestion.

Sweeteners and Sugar Alcohols

Sweeteners like sorbitol, erythritol, xylitol, and mannitol cannot be fully digested by many people and result in bloating, gas, and other ill health effects. Monk fruit sweetener or Stevia have been shown to be better options.

Sodas and Other Carbonated Drinks

Did you know that sodas and other fizzy drinks can cause gas and bloating?

Why? Because they significantly increase the amount of air you swallow when you drink! The bubbles in carbonated drinks are actually gas that gets trapped in your stomach. They can create the sensation of helium being pumped into your stomach (like a balloon). That's why we feel bloated when we drink carbonated beverages. In fact, any carbonated drink, even sparking water, can cause bloating.

Of course, when air is swallowed into the digestive tract, it has to be passed—*one way or the other.* To avoid this, drink something else instead, like tea, water, or any non-carbonated, low sugar juice! Try coconut water or a fresh-squeezed lemonade with mint and slices of strawberry, instead!

And while clean, fresh, uncarbonated water is good for us, research has also shown that even drinking *too much water all at once* can cause bloating because it dilutes the digestive juices in our guts. Pace yourself.

In addition to the gas you put into your stomach when you drink soda, there might be any number of ingredients in there that you should avoid: artificial sweeteners, sugar, flavorings, and dyes are a few.

It is also important to note that, on average, a twelve ounce can of soda provides as many as 150 calories, in addition to forty to fifty grams of high fructose corn syrup. That's the equivalent of ten teaspoons of sugar. Yes, you read it right. TEN TEA-SPOONS OF SUGAR! Nutritional experts have pointed out that drinking just one can of soda per day, without reducing the intake of high fructose corn syrup from other sources, can lead to a weight gain of 15 lb. in one year!

Chewing Gum

Bummer, I know. It's the go-to quick fix for bad breath, especially when you are about to land that French kiss on your object of desire. But you probably didn't know that by chewing that same breath-freshening gum, you may have to cut the cheese at an inopportune moment! Yes, folks, chewing gum can make you swallow more air than usual and thus make you bloated.

To make matters worse, many of the "sugar-free" gums available in the market are sweetened with hard-to-digest sugar alcohols, like sorbitol, mannitol, and xylitol. That is one of the reasons why, as part of my protocol to stop excessive burping, I tell my patients to stop chewing gum. Avoiding chewing gum will reduce excessive gas in the gut.

Processed Foods

"If it didn't grow that way, don't eat it."
—E. de Mello, MD, PhD

"Duh!" you say. You'd think that avoiding processed foods was common knowledge by now. But many people don't know that this junk food category, besides the obvious snack foods, also includes most cereals, breads, and even salad dressings. All of these foods tend to contain fructose, lactose and a lot of other junk. If your goal is to stop the annoying, excessive bloating and gas, start by saying, "Hell no!" to processed foods. Steer clear of all processed foods and anything else that contains additives. If you don't recognize something in the ingredient list by its name, it is likely an additive.

Processed foods are also loaded with added sugar and salt, resulting in dehydration. These foods pull water into the body rather than out, which in turn may result in more bloating.

Food Dye = Food Danger!

No wonder they're called *dyes*. As you eat them, you slowly die!

Food dyes are usually listed as colors and numbers, such as Blue 1, Blue 2, Green 3, Red 3, Red 40, Yellow 5, Yellow 6. In sensitive children, these dyes have been shown to contribute to ADHD. In fact, the FDA determined in the eighties that Red Dye #3 was a carcinogen. However, surprise, surprise, the food industry lobby put pressure on the agency and eventually succeeded in preventing the crimson culprit from being banned.

High levels of the carcinogenic *benzedrine food coloring* in the Yellow 5 and 6 dyes were reported by a study in the 1990s and yet, these dyes remain in our foods.[8] Conversion of benzedrine to its amphetamine acid form also gave color to the once very popular "congo red" dye. Benzedrine and its derived amphetamines have been used as stimulants throughout the years, and you don't really want them coloring your food.[9]

Often used with artificial flavorings to simulate the look and taste of specific real foods such as fruit, eggs, meats, or vegetables, the use of dyes in foods has grown exponentially. Year after year, the food industry creates more and more "tasty junk" to lure us into their greedy web.

Hard Candy

Similar to drinking carbonated drinks, sucking on hard candy means swallowing extra air. Those of us with kids at home can relate. Little kids do plant stink-bombs after eating hard candy!

In addition, some candy manufacturers use sorbitol as a sweetener, which can contribute to extra gas.

High Fructose Corn Syrup

This starchy, sweet syrup is an additive in thousands and thousands of processed foods—many of which you would never suspect. We know that High Fructose Corn Syrup (HFCS) causes insulin resistance. If not corrected, it will probably lead to obesity and type 2 diabetes. Consuming HFCS changes how our blood flows through our brain. It also alters one's liver enzyme profile, leading to both acute and chronic subclinical inflammation. *Subclinical* means "below the clinical threshold" (so there is no way to technically measure and know the reason why you feel so horrible).

Read the ingredients on the label!

Nutrition Facts

12 servings per container
Serving size 12 fl oz (360 mL)

Amount per serving
Calories 150

	% DV*
Total Fat 0g	**0%**
Sodium 30mg	**1%**
Total Carbohydrate 41g	**15%**
Total Sugars 41g	
Includes 41g Added Sugars	**83%**
Protein 0g	

Not a significant source of other nutrients.

* % DV = % Daily Value

CARBONATED WATER, HIGH FRUCTOSE CORN SYRUP, CARAMEL COLOR, SUGAR, PHOSPHORIC ACID, CAFFEINE, CITRIC ACID, NATURAL FLAVOR. SEE UNIT CONTAINER FOR MANUFACTURER'S IDENTITY.

Oh look . . . there's "high-fructose corn syrup" near the top of the list! This means it's a main ingredient! Did you know that **ingredients are listed in the order of their predominance in the product,** from highest to lowest? The ingredient listed first on the package is the thing there is most of in that product. The ingredients are listed in descending order of quantity.

Did you know your body produces a hormone that controls hunger and satiation? Often referred to as the "satiety hormone" or the "starvation hormone," leptin is produced and released by fat cells, and it helps regulate our body weight. When fat mass increases, leptin levels and our appetite are supposed to be suppressed, and energy intake, hopefully, optimally controlled.

But high fructose corn syrup blocks all of that from happening. As a result, we don't realize we have eaten enough! Then, we overeat and feel bloated.

Using *high fructose corn syrup* in place of cane sugars in soda and other sweetened drinks made them *cheaper* and more easily accessible to everyone, including low-income families. These are the same families who, at least in the United States, are disproportionally obese. Soon after the introduction of HFCS in soft drinks, "super-sized" portions were also introduced, contributing further to the epidemic of preventable ailments, including bloating, diabetes, and heart disease.

Fructose (the "F" in HFCS) is metabolized differently than glucose. While glucose is transported into the cells of the body by the hormone *insulin*, fructose is not. Eating fructose does not stimulate insulin release, which is essential for proper metabolism and digestion. Specifically, fructose ingestion does not stimulate the body to produce leptin, a vital hormone that tells the body when we are "full" or "satiated" after we eat. Consuming excessive amounts of fructose leads to leptin resistance, meaning you don't feel satiated after a fructose-rich meal, which in turn leads you to eat more. Leptin resistance combined with the typical high-fat, high-calorie diet has significantly contributed to the current obesity epidemic in the U.S. and many other parts of the world.

Besides aggravating digestive problems, a high-fructose diet can also lead to an elevated risk of high blood pressure, stroke, and pre-diabetes (also known as "metabolic syndrome.")

How Did High Fructose Corn Syrup End Up in Our food?

The good ol' 70s is to blame again! And you thought bell bottoms were bad! Wait till you hear this . . . HFCS is present in most fast foods. From sodas, to ketchup, to cereals, to salad dressings, this ingredient is everywhere. The sad news is that HFCS is probably here to stay.

In fact, high fructose corn syrups have been the darling of the processed food industry in the United States and, by default, the rest of the world. Many condiments are known to contain sugars, but they often have fancy and difficult-to-pronounce names to purposefully trick the consumer into thinking they are buying something "healthy and sugar-free."

When reading food labels, look for words ending in "ose" such as in" fructose." This word has "fruct" in it (just one letter off from "fruit"). It almost sounds healthy, doesn't it? But, it is no accident that this word makes you think of the word "fruit." Fructose is an all-time junk food ingredient that can be a health risk to many of us.

How to Get a Leg on Up on Your Bloating and Gas

We will delve into this further in chapter nine: Treatment. But for now . . .

1. Eliminate the trigger foods we have discussed, then gradually re-introduce them one by one. Keep a daily

food journal to see if your symptoms return after reintroducing the trigger foods.
2. Consider adding a probiotic and a digestive enzyme to your daily regimen.
3. Exercise and increase sweating. It will help your body eliminate the toxins through your largest organ, your skin.

Have you heard of *activated charcoal underwear?* While you are trying to determine the cause of your bloating, and for those whose "bad wind" will not stop, no matter what, activated charcoal underwear—featuring fabulous fart-filtering fabrics that trap and neutralize your stink bombs—can be a good temporary solution!

CHAPTER

6

Food Labels: What to Consume

"You are what you eat and have been fed."

—Unknown

We have all heard scary stories about the dangers of hidden ingredients lurking in processed foods. Like the mother who thought she was buying a healthy snack for her child—but the snack contained peanuts, masquerading as something else. It wasn't clearly indicated on the label, and her son was allergic. This led to a terrifying trip to the ER and unnecessary medical bills.

For some, consuming certain "hidden" ingredients is life threatening, and it has happened to so many people because even when they read the labels, they still *did not really know what they were eating*!

So, here is some background information that I hope is useful in learning to read food labels.

The Tiger Has A New Cage

Chile is a relatively small South American country with a population of about nineteen million. The United States has roughly seventeen times that many people, but Chile still leads the global fight for consumer-friendly food labeling!

Several years back, *Forbes* magazine ranked Chile as one of the "fattest" countries in the world, with 65.3% of its citizens having an unhealthy body weight.[1] By 2016, Chilean health officials had become extremely concerned with the growing threat of obesity, and its associated health problems (and even deaths). One Chilean citizen was dying every hour from obesity, and the government saw better food labeling as the first step in remedying the dilemma. They decided to wage an all-out war on unhealthy foods by employing and enforcing strict marketing regulations and mandatory packaging redesigns, based on clear labeling rules.

As one example, the smiling, friendly tiger on the box of Frosted Flakes®, an American brand of cereal made by General Mills®, was replaced with plain boxes with no cartoon tiger, and it had to identify the product as high in sugar and calories.

This mandatory packaging standard instituted in Chile is considered to be the most ambitious attempt to remake a country's food culture by experts in the nutritional field.[2] They may become the model for adequately addressing the global obesity epidemic that, according to the World Health Organization, is a disaster in the making.

Chile's ambitious goal is to help stop the train wreck by preventing four million premature deaths a year. According to Chilean government officials, the opinions of the food industry were considered, but the policies were crafted to put the people's health as the first priority, ahead of the interests of the food industry.

They started with the premise that most people's shopping habits don't include reading every label. After all, who has time? It's a grab-and-go, baby! So, Chile's Ministry of Health hired graphic designers to develop easy-to-see (and read) warning labels. *Black-and-white stop signs* were created to identify products with an excessive quantity of sugar, calories, salt or fat. The marketing campaign slogan was "Choose foods with fewer signs, and if they don't have any, even better."

Now, noticeable, clear labels describe products as "High in Sugar," "High in Calories," "High in Fat," and "High in Salt," so people know what they are buying. That helps.

Food Labeling, Politics, and Money in the U.S.

After decades of hard-to-follow nutritional recommendations and misleading health claims on so many food packages, the Food and Drug Administration (FDA) finally caved to public pressure. Starting in the late 1990s, the FDA required food companies to include "Nutrition Fact" labels on all products. This included information about sugar, protein, fats, carbohydrates, and sodium content, as well as some vitamin and mineral information.

This was followed by the 2006 "Food Allergen Labeling and Consumer Protection Act" that required food packaging to identify ingredients more clearly. Instead of misleading the public with terms that are difficult to recognize, the food industry was required to identify ingredients in simple terms.

Take casein, for example. Casein is a milk-derived protein. If you are lactose intolerant, you need to know it's in there. Now every packaged food such as potato chips, cookies, and even "healthy foods" such as granola bars, must list its contents in plain language if they contain potential allergens.

Peanuts contain one of the most common and dangerous food allergens. For some, consuming them can lead to death. Because of concerns about allergies and potential anaphylactic shock, most airlines have eliminated serving them. Some schools have banned peanuts or their derivative products altogether. Now, packaging must clearly state if a product contains any sign of peanuts. These "May Contain . . ." warnings will also warn when foods are produced somewhere where any cross-contamination is possible, even though a product may not actually have peanuts listed as an ingredient.

"Why Did This Have to Happen?"

From a Facebook posting, whose author asked that this story be shared everywhere to help others.
July 12, 2018

Our hearts are broken and we are still in shock. Our whole lives we dedicated to keeping our child safe from one ingredient: peanuts.

On Monday, June 25, our 15-year-old daughter, *Jane Doe* (name changed for confidentiality), while at a friend's house, made a fatal choice. There was an open package of Chips Ahoy cookies, the top flap of the package was pulled back, and the packaging was too similar to what we had previously deemed "safe" to her. She ate one cookie of chewy Chips Ahoy thinking it was safe because of the "red" packaging, only to find out too late that there was an added ingredient . . . Reese's peanut butter cups/ chips. She started feeling tingling in her mouth and came straight home. Her condition rapidly deteriorated. She went into anaphylactic shock, stopped breathing, and went unconscious. We administered two epi-pens while she was conscious and waited on paramedics for what felt like an eternity.

She died within one and a half hours of eating the cookie.

As a mother who diligently taught her the ropes of what was okay to ingest and what was not, I feel lost and angry because she knew her limits and was aware of familiar packaging. She knew what "safe" was. A small added indication on the pulled-back flap on a familiar red package wasn't enough to call out to her that there was "peanut product" in the cookies before it was too late. I want to share our story with everyone because we want to spread awareness. The company has different colored packaging to indicate chunky, chewy, or regular, but NO screaming warnings about such a fatal ingredient to many people. Especially children.

It's important to us to spread awareness so that this horrible mistake doesn't happen again. Please share.

The Food Industry's Relentless Opposition to Food Labeling

Despite strong scientific evidence showing that food labels do help consumers make healthier choices, the food industry is still making misleading claims to the contrary.

Food Company Tactics

The food industry uses a variety of tactics to mislead the public. Many food companies argue that labeling confuses consumers, even though no significant scientific studies support this argument.

Questioning the Science

When studies showed that "added sugar" information on labels helps consumers make more appropriate choices, the food industry spent a significant amount of money in an attempt to discredit the studies, trying to add doubt by arguing that consumers would interpret the information incorrectly.

Publishing Biased Studies

A study by the International Food Information Council concluded that the added sugars disclosure line would be "misleading" to consumers.[3] The problem was that the study did not provide respondents' information completely enough to evaluate their food purchases accurately.

Avoidance

The food industry is known for diverting attention from scientific evidence by making unsubstantiated claims about how labeling will affect consumer thinking. The maker of Campbell's Soup went so far as to suggest that the added sugars line would "confuse consumers by taking their focus off of calories."[4]

Consumers Fight Back

Several consumer advocacy groups raised class action lawsuits accusing General Mills, maker of Nature Valley granola bars, of deceptive packaging. Their granola bars, the lawsuits contended, were not "100% natural" because they contained not only processed ingredients, like corn syrup and the additive maltodextrin, but also the pesticide glyphosate, which is a carcinogen known to be harmful to humans.

The suits demanded that General Mills remove the words "100% natural" from its granola bar labels. General Mills fought back, saying "We stand behind our products and the accuracy of our labels." The company then agreed to remove the "100% natural" claim from its packaging, which now reads "made with 100% natural oats."[5] Aren't all oats natural?

A Hard-to-Swallow Truth

The food industry lobby exerts an overwhelming influence on food labeling standards. They have attempted and have successfully blocked almost all new legislation on the issue. For example, the requirement that added sugars be included under "Nutritional Facts" came only after decades of lobbying by public interest groups.

The Sugar Association, representing 142,000 growers,

processors, and distributors, was initially vehemently opposed to the new rule, arguing that "metabolically, your cells don't know if the sugar came from an apple or a gummy bear." While the statement is half true, apples have useful vitamins and fiber, while a gummy bear has neither. Also, the gummy probably uses different chemicals as food coloring, too. Hardly the same as an apple!

The hard truth is that hiding food ingredients, especially chemicals proven to be dangerous and sometimes carcinogenic, is a well-known, very blunt deception employed by much of the food industry.

And apparently, they do it legally.

You should know that almost everything that is commercialized has sugar in it. Masquerading as "sugar-free," sugar alcohols like xylitol, mannitol, and sorbitol contain the problematic FODMAP properties discussed in previous chapters. Commercial foods, especially those with high fructose corn syrup, lead to bloating because our GI system cannot readily digest these artificial ingredients.

READ THOSE LABELS!

Opt for cleaner versions of products that contain as few additives or dyes as possible. And watch for hidden sources of sugars. Eat whole foods as much as possible. A "whole food" is one that is in its unadulterated, natural state—not processed or broken down. It is less likely to be in a package. If it comes in a box, it is more likely that the food has been processed.

As I explained in the microbiome chapter, the colon is home to trillions of different bacteria. Most bacteria in the colon are there to help the gastrointestinal system break down and metabolize the foods we eat. We, the host, and they, the helpers, both rely on what we eat in order to thrive. Remember that certain foods are more likely to cause bad bacteria to grow and even sometimes overtake the good bacteria.

The Kid with a Severe Sugar Allergy

Maria, a precocious fourteen-year-old, has known the importance of reading food labels ever since she can remember. Maria has a severe sensitivity to sugars of all kinds. Although a true allergy to sugar is very rare, intolerances are quite common.

Maria wanted to feel that she belonged and was accepted by her peers. She didn't want to be regarded as "weird or freaky" and be cast aside at her new high school. So, Maria decided that she was no longer going to read every single packaged food label when it was offered to her. "Not in this new school," she told me.

She did not discuss her decision with her parents or the school nurse. Her parents had taken the precaution of briefing the nurse of the significant symptoms that resulted when Maria ingested almost anything containing sugar. The only exceptions were apple or coconut sugar.

And so, when Edward—the cute boy she met during freshman orientation—offered her a "sugar-free" gummy bear, Maria played it cool and accepted it, as a way to connect with him. She did ask him before eating it, "What does 'sugar-free' mean? Are they artificially sweetened?" Edward answered, "No. It's sweetened with fruit juice, like apple juice, but not the bad stuff. I don't do well when I eat regular sugar," he said.

Maria felt quietly excited. After all, she may have more in common with her new crush than she'd thought! "Well, that's very interesting," she said. Maria felt safe because Edward was also conscientious about choosing sugar-free foods. So, she ate the gummy bear that was already in her hand, then she reached inside the package for another one.

Not twenty minutes later, Maria realized she was in deep trouble. She first started feeling nauseous and extremely tired; then she got severe abdominal cramps, followed by painful bloating and gas. She wiped her forehead when she started sweating, but said nothing to either Edward or the teacher.

All of a sudden, Maria had an overwhelming urge to go to the bathroom. Unfortunately, she didn't make it in time. She vomited right there in the hallway, and then got diarrhea. Terrified and filled with shame, Maria asked the nurse to call her mother to come to pick her up. She couldn't face going to school for the rest of that week.

What was listed in the package of gummy bears?

Under "natural" flavors, it listed Lycasin, which contains maltitol, a sugar alcohol that is almost as sweet as table sugar but half as caloric. The brand of gummy bear that Edward had was Haribo. The Amazon.com description for sugar-free Haribo Gummy Bears reads in part: "This product is a sugarless/sugar-free item with ingredients that can cause intestinal distress if eaten in excess."

How, when, and why did reading food labels become so challenging?

It seems that knowing what food labels mean almost requires a master's degree. Packaged food labels have always been complicated because these products are filled with complicated ingredients, and, with dollar signs on its mind, the food industry has little concern for our safety. The claims that the food industry has been making about what is in our food are out of control.

Hard-to-pronounce chemicals are not the only issue, either. We can no longer take at face value the words that are used to describe a package's contents.

Understanding Food Description Labels

From "organic" produce, to "USDA-inspected" meat, to "cage-free" eggs and "pesticide-free" whatever else, understanding what is and is not in the food we eat can be a little overwhelming.

The main problems persist due to ineffective regulation by the FDA and relentless lobbying by the food industry. Many food manufacturers do not want you to know that they are manipulating your taste buds to get you hooked on their food. The result is that you are often left wondering what the truth really is, leading to more and more confusion as consumers try to make sense of the array of information and misinformation.

It is true that we all need safe food and drinking water; we need to know where it comes from and what is in it. That is our basic right. But the existing food labeling rules are vague. No legislation requires food companies to give us the information we want to know. For example, the food industry often challenges legislation that attempts to differentiate between foods that are produced by "sustainable" farms that are using humane practices and those produced by large corporate agribusinesses, "green-washing" their products to make them look more friendly.

It seems that the more we attempt to eat healthier, the more the food industry manipulates the information they give the consumer about what exactly is in our food.

So, let's break down what the labels mean:

Certified Organic

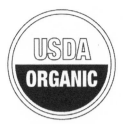

The U.S. Department of Agriculture (USDA) organic seal is a registered trademark, and if it is on your food, it means that specific government standards have been met:

- Organic crops cannot be grown with synthetic fertilizers, synthetic pesticides, or sewage sludge.
- Organic crops cannot be genetically modified (GMO) or irradiated.
- Animals must eat only organically grown feed (without animal byproducts) and can't be treated with synthetic hormones or antibiotics at any time.
- Organically raised animals must have access to the outdoors, and ruminants (hoofed animals, including cows) must have access to pasture.
- Animals cannot be cloned.

Country of Origin Label

Currently, the USDA requires Country of Origin Labeling (COOL) for some foods, but not all. For example, foods such as chicken, seafood, produce and some nuts provide necessary information about the country these foods came from, but transparency is still somewhat lacking.

Here is how the food industry gets its way in Congress. Beef and pork were covered by mandatory "country of origin" labeling rules until 2015, when the meat industry pressured Congress to repeal this labeling requirement. What this means is that when you buy commercial beef and pork, you have no idea where it came from or the country of origin's practice for raising and slaughtering these animals. This exemplifies why the labeling of meat is often under question and how the food industry usually wins and we lose.

When I looked into how other countries do this, I found out that most developed countries (including Japan, China, Australia, even Russia and some countries with emerging economies, like Brazil) require that country of origin information be provided on meat packaging. Many of these countries' governments also require food producers to label products that contain GMO ingredients. These exact requirements change from time to time, though, based on evolving trade agreements.

USDA Inspected

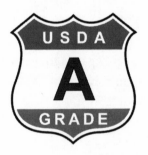

The USDA seal is placed on food that has met established quality standards and is ranked by its quality. "USDA Grade A" beef or eggs, for example, are graded *based on quality and size* but not for how they are raised. In other words, the USDA seal tells the consumer nothing about the producing company's practices or the quality of life of the animal. The majority of the meats in grocery stores have a USDA seal of inspection. Otherwise, they are not supposed to be sold to the public.

Cage-Free Eggs

"Cage-free" refers to birds that are not raised in constricting cages, without saying anything about the other living conditions the chickens may face. For instance, eggs that are legally labeled as "cage-free" could still come from birds raised indoors in overcrowded spaces at large, poorly ventilated factory farms.

Hormone Free

Federal law prohibits the use of hormones given to hogs and poultry. The use of the term "hormone-free" on pork and poultry products is intended to mislead the consumer into paying a higher price for the product. As for dairy products, "hormone free" refers to milk with no added hormones that comes from cows not treated with rBGH.

Seafood Labels: Farm Raised vs. Wild Caught

Seafood labels are often misleading. Organic labels on fish are deceiving because there is no U.S. government standard for organic seafood certification. Additionally, you may see labels like "farm-raised" and "wild caught" on your seafood.

"Farm-raised" tuna, salmon, shrimp, clams (or any other fish) were raised in an enclosed pen; probably one submerged in a pond, lake, or salt water. Alternatively, "Wild Caught" fish and seafood live a natural life spent entirely in the ocean, lake, river, or stream of their origin, and have been captured by a fisherman (or woman). I recommend these.

Free Range

"Free Range" labels are regulated by the USDA and are only used for poultry and not for pigs, cattle, or egg-producing chickens. "Free Range" can be used even if the chicken had minimal outdoor access. So how *free* is the range? This label does not really say if the animal was ever actually allowed outdoors to roam freely.

Natural and Naturally

Meat and poultry products that are "Raised Naturally," according to USDA rules, cannot contain artificial colors, artificial flavors, preservatives, or other artificial ingredients. But other labels like "natural" or "minimally processed" are meaningless because they do not tell the consumer what the animals were fed, how they were raised, or if antibiotics or hormones were used. When you see "natural" on the label, there might be very little you would actually find natural about the product inside.

Fresh vs. Frozen

The official label "fresh" is used only on poultry and means that the meat was not cooled below 26 degrees. It is good to remember that poultry does not have to be labeled as "frozen" until it reaches zero degrees Fahrenheit. *Wow.* When we see the word "fresh," we don't think of frozen, processed, or preserved. But the FDA allows this misleading practice to flourish and consumers are led to believe that the poultry they are purchasing has not been frozen, processed, or preserved in any way. The USDA does not define or regulate the use of the "fresh" label on any other type of products.

GMO Labels

A variety of the processed foods today contain genetically engineered ingredients. But what does GMO really mean? GMO, or *genetically modified*, means that the whole food or other ingredients used to make a particular food product are altered at the genetic level. Usually by adding genetic material from a different species, or by making other changes that couldn't happen through traditional, classical breeding. There is no scientific consensus regarding the safety of these foods. And often, the approval process for a new GMO crop relies on testing that is done by the very companies that are selling these genetically engineered foods to us. In July 2016, Congress went against what 90% of

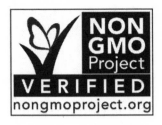

Americans said they wanted, passing a federal law *blocking* states from requiring GMO labeling. This new federal law overturned existing state laws that did require clear GMO labeling, and instead allowed for GMO foods to be labeled with 800-numbers or QR codes, directing people to do their own research about what they are eating. While it's good to know where to look for more information, this is not a good substitute for clear labels on packaged foods.

Grass-Fed, or Grass Finished

"Grass-fed" is supposed to mean that an animal's main source of food comes from grass or foliage and not from corn or grains. But much of the "grass-fed" meat you see in stores today was "grain-finished," meaning that after it reached maturity it was fed a diet that included grains and other things that are definitely not grass (like potatoes, beets, and hay). Animal farming companies submit their own (unsubstantiated) standards to the USDA so they can put a "grass-fed" claim on their products. They are able to do so because there are no government regulations for this labeling.

No Antibiotics

Large-scale producers are known to feed animals antibiotics at low doses to promote growth, improve feed efficiency, and prevent disease. "No antibiotics" on the label is supposed to mean that no antibiotics were ever used over an animal's lifetime: not by injection, not in food, not in their water, nowhere. We already know that the terrifying public health threat of antibiotic-resistant bacteria is, at least in part, caused by overuse of antibiotics, particularly in our meat and poultry industries. Some producers say that not using any antibiotics threatens the entire herd population, and so they get away with using antibiotics only to treat sick animals. But they can still say the products produced from those animals have no antibiotics if there is a long enough "clean" time after the administration of the antibiotics and the animal's ultimate demise. Luckily, the term "certified organic" cannot be used if antibiotics have been used at any time. If an animal has been given antibiotics for any reason, its meat, milk, or eggs cannot be labeled as organic.

No Added Hormones vs. Hormone Free

Animals (and even vegetables) have hormones naturally. "Raised without added hormones," or "no hormones administered," or "no synthetic hormones" means that no *synthetic* hormones were fed to them. Synthetic hormones are "synthesized" from the hormones of pregnant animals, mostly horses. However, "hormone-free" labels do not disclose what else the animals were fed or if they were given antibiotics.

Is My Food Treated With Radiation?

Irradiated foods are everywhere. This topic deserves its own chapter, but let me give you a quick history on the subject.

Irradiation, also called "cold" pasteurization, is the process whereby food is exposed to a controlled amount of "ionizing radiation." This is done using either Gamma rays, X-rays, or electron beam radiation. The intent is to kill harmful bacteria like salmonella and e. Coli in order to prevent spoilage and increase shelf life.

Federal law states that all irradiated foods that are sold in grocery stores must be labeled and marked with the Radura

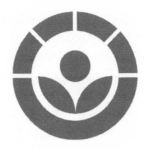

symbol. This, however, does not apply to restaurants, schools, or hospitals!

In theory, irradiation makes sense—making food safer for consumption is a vital part of public health—but opponents argue that subjecting food to radiation has potential side effects and does more harm than good. In addition, they argue that radiation is not even an effective way to prevent disease or food spoilage. Some go so far as to say that irradiating foods may actually be spawning radiation-resistant forms of bacteria and other potential health risks.

"Irradiation is being embraced by the food industry as a way to mask filthy conditions in factory-style slaughterhouses and processing plants. Because it greatly extends the shelf life of food, irradiation is also being embraced by multinational corporations as a way to move food production operations to developing nations, a trend that has already financially imperiled multitudes of American farmers and ranchers."[6]

Is Food Irradiation Really Dangerous?

The World Health Organization and the U.S. Department of Agriculture both insist that food irradiation is safe and that it eliminates dangerous bacteria in human food, while also preventing the spread of disease in livestock, by providing cleaner, safer (irradiated) feed. Several national and international studies have concluded that food irradiation is safe and even vital for food safety. They say irradiating food does not take away or "steal" nutrients from foods and, when used properly, can help prevent the food-borne illnesses that affect an estimated 48 million people (one in six Americans) per year, killing about 3,000.[7]

Groups that don't want to see our food supply subjected to radiation, like Food and Water Watch, have strongly lobbied against the technique. They argue that it might lead manufacturers to "zap" food instead of maintaining a clean plant.

The thought is that food irradiation facilitates faster line speeds at meat facilities and allows plant workers to get away with sloppier handling practices. Microbiologists argue that, even when irradiated, if a food facility plant is dirty, understaffed, poorly inspected, or not following well-established safety standards, the food is still going to be bad. Food irradiation, while it may eliminate some microorganisms and even insects, will not be able to fix everything.

Remember, not all bacteria is bad bacteria. Studies show that 95% of crucial bacteria is killed during the irradiation process, meaning we are killing the good bacteria that help us digest our food along with the ones that make food spoil.

When food goes bad, those bacteria give off a bad smell, alerting us that we should not eat it. Irradiation can make what should look like old, rotten food look and feel fresh,[8] allowing the food industry to continue to make a profit at the expense of unwitting consumers.

In the United States, many foods have been approved for irradiation, including:

- Beef and pork
- Poultry
- Molluscan shellfish (e.g., oysters, clams, mussels, and scallops)
- Shell eggs
- Fresh fruits and vegetables

- Lettuce and spinach
- Spices and seasonings
- Seeds for sprouting (e.g., for alfalfa sprouts)

What About Organic Foods? . . . Are They Irradiated?

In the U.S., all irradiated foods must be labeled as such, *except* for "multi-ingredient" foods—anything with more than one ingredient.

It is very hard to know which packaged foods that contain more than one ingredient (i.e., almost all packaged foods) have been irradiated or not. Any one of the ingredients in your favorite spice mix may have been irradiated—and they don't even have to tell you. Buy organic as often as possible if you choose to avoid eating irradiated food.

CHAPTER
7

The Three Amigos:
Our Three Brains

"In most cases, dysfunction in our bodies is the result of an imbalance of the three brains."

—E. de Mello, MD, PhD

No, you do not need new reading glasses. You heard it right. We have three brains! We have already talked about the *second* brain (the gut!). But *three* brains? Most people think, I can barely handle the one in my head!

Yes, the first and obvious one is the HEAD, then there's the second brain, the GUT. But there's also the HEART brain. These three interconnected brains function via an extensive network of neurons, each having particular roles. When in balance, these connections and their collective information highway provide stability, grounding, and the ability to use intuition (gut feelings) to create ultimate health. The gut brain alone contains about one hundred million neurons and works independently of—and in conjunction with—the head and heart brains.

As discussed, research has shown that gut bacteria (the microbiota) directly communicate with the head brain and play a critical role in mood, memory, and cognition, as well as in recognizing feelings of satiation.

Anxiety and depression, for example, are conditions that

we know contribute to gastrointestinal conditions, such as IBS, SIBO, and "Leaky Gut"—all of which present with bloating as a common denominator.

The gut feeling (intuition) or "butterflies in the stomach" that you get when you have to make a decision about something important is actually a physiological response to signals from our head to our gut. This "little brain hidden in our gut" has revolutionized our understanding of the link between overall health, digestion, and elimination.

The Three Brains and How They Relate To One Another

The Three Brain connection goes all the way back to the beginning of life when we were but a few small cells in our mother's womb. The ENS (enteric nervous system) is the very first system to develop in our body, and it is hardwired into our gut. It plays a very important role. Signals between the ENS and the gut control secretions and blood flow, allowing us to efficiently digest and absorb our food.

Chronic inflammation is now known to be the leading cause of many chronic diseases we face today, including bloating, heart disease, and even cancer.

The Three Brains: Their Distinct and Combined Roles

The human brain has survived and adapted to the many challenges it's encountered since the beginning of time. Continually evolving and improving its impressive array of tasks, it has resulted in the magnificent and powerful machine that we have today.

The initial brain, originally primitive in nature, was focused on survival and adaptation. It developed over time, through many complex and distinct stages, into what we know today as the three-pound organ that controls and dictates all that we do to operate effectively.

Working together, the head, heart, and gut brains play distinct, vital roles:

1. The Head brain analyzes and applies logic.
2. The Heart brain senses the world of emotions and feelings.
3. The Gut brain teaches us self-preservation by directing us to follow our instinct, the "gut feelings" we all have the ability to experience.

These three amigos help us to understand our identity and who we are in the world.

CASE STUDY

The "Atypical" Diagnosis for a Typical Patient in Denial

Josh, a 43-year-old executive, had received a diagnosis of *atypical ulcerative colitis* from an ER physician. This is a debilitating and compromising immune condition. In Josh's case, abdominal pain and the diarrhea that followed were among his most irritating symptoms.

Josh often threw up at work and had significant stomach discomfort such as nausea, diarrhea, and way too many visits to the bathroom in a short window of time.

For clarification, the word "atypical" is often placed in front of a diagnosis when the symptoms substantially differ from the usual presentation of the disease. Furthermore, a biopsy must confirm a diagnosis of ulcerative colitis. In Josh's case, no diagnosis followed to confirm this condition. Plus, he was not presenting with one of the cardinal signs of ulcerative colitis—blood in the stool.

The first thing I noticed when Josh and his wife showed up at my office was a reluctance on Josh's part to take his condition seriously. He casually attributed his symptoms to being overly stressed at work.

He went on, "You know what, I can deal with this on my own. I bet if I were to ignore it, it would eventually go away, all by itself."

Josh's wife, Anabel, who was clearly more concerned than he was, said that Josh had made an appointment to see me a year before, but he had canceled it.

Josh cut in, "Honestly, Doc, I was too busy and had no time for this crap, literally and figuratively."

He rolled his eyes as his wife went on. "One time his abdominal pain, gas, and nausea got so bad that I insisted on taking his blood pressure—I used to be a nurse's assistant. It was 180 over 110. I'm sure you know the average normal is 120 over 80! His heart rate was sky high. He couldn't stop vomiting. So, I called 911!"

Josh took over telling the story. "She was afraid both my heart and gut would literally blow up."

They went on, trading descriptions:

ANABEL: As usual, he was extremely bloated and
    passing an abundance of *very* foul, stinky gas.
JOSH: I was so embarrassed in the ER, Doc.
ANABEL: After asking only two or three questions, the
    ER doctor decided that Josh's had *ulcerative colitis*.
JOSH: She said I needed to go on steroids and see a

surgeon because in most cases, part of the colon has
to be removed.

ANABEL: She never asked about his diet—which was
horrible—or his stress level . . .

JOSH: . . . which is through the roof! Sleep and exercise
are luxuries I cannot afford . . .

ANABEL: . . . in his quest to become more and more
successful.

JOSH: The ER doc's diagnosis left me literally numb.
Some surgeon's going to have to remove part of my
colon? And I'll likely need to wear a colostomy bag
for a few months? How will I be able to work?

Anabel shook her head in frustration. "WORK? *That's* the
first thing that came to your mind?!"

So why was Josh, Mr. Obstinate, even here? Anabel had
called my office from the ER and pleaded with my staff to
get her husband in, a.s.a.p., or he was going to "drive himself
into the ground with this new diagnosis."

The first thing that struck me about Josh was his inability
to connect with his body and the symptoms. The ER diagnosis was just a big bother to him. "I have no time for this,
Dr. de Mello."

When I asked him what he thought was the trigger for
his condition, he shrugged and said, "Oh Doc, I just need to
find a better assistant to help me at work, and then all will
be fine." Josh's denial about what he was doing to his body,
coupled with his ability to completely ignore his body's cries
for help, was astounding.

I dug further. "I see," I said, "but if this misdiagnosed condition had a voice, what would it say to you?" He struggled
to understand the meaning of my question, then mumbled,
"Well, maybe I am a little too stressed out."

I asked Josh if he was ready to do the work necessary to avoid surgery. "You'll need to dedicate a significant amount of time to doing labs, change your diet, sleep at least seven hours a night, exercise regularly." Here's where I almost lost him. "Listen to your body, Josh. It's talking to you. The symptoms are your body's language—saying to you that things are off, causing you to be dis-EASED—and that you've been a pretty negligent father to your body."

He looked a little wounded, so I added, "I'm not saying this is all your fault—there's a disconnect between your three brains, Josh." He shot me a confused look, so I continued, counting to three with my fingers as I spoke, "Your traditional *head* brain, your *gut* brain and your *heart* brain."

Blessedly, Anabel insisted that Josh take a month off work. He hadn't taken any personal time in over three years. After meeting with the functional nutritionist in my office, they decided to hire a cook to prepare their meals three times a week. Josh joined a neighborhood gym. Anabel took him to her meditation class, which, at first, he described as "a big waste of time." But only four weeks later he admitted, "Now I am totally hooked!"

Next, we talked about his issues with an herbal protocol for his condition. We also addressed the overgrowth of Candida and his reliance on protein bars three times a day for energy boosts. These bars are usually loaded with sugar and are "food bombs." They may look good, but they'll blow you up (bloat). Josh's lifestyle changes included removing all added sugars from his diet and most fruits, except for blueberries, blackberries and green apples.

At Josh's thirty-day follow-up appointment, he reported feeling about 25% better, but he was still not convinced that he could refrain from going back to "doing his life" the way he had for all these years. Like an alcoholic in denial, Josh felt that it would be okay if once in a while he missed getting a good night's sleep, maybe ate a couple helpings of fried food—"I *love* them, Doc!"—and had a few drinks, which leads to smoking a few cigarettes with his work buddies. All this after a twelve- to fourteen-hour work shift.

"Don't get me wrong, Doc. I'll do most of what you're suggesting," he winked conspiratorially, "but I can't commit to these changes for the rest of my life."

"Well, I see, Josh," I replied. "It sounds like you made the decision then that surgery is your preferred option." He didn't back down. He gave a shoulder shrug and casually said, "Well, maybe it is, Doc."

"Okay Josh," I said, just as nonchalantly. "But do you realize that for your symptoms to permanently go away—even after surgery—you'll still need to change your lifestyle?"

Josh looked like a deer in the headlights; he did not see that coming. He had not considered this scenario. I pressed on, "You have SIBO and Candida overgrowth, Josh, not ulcerative colitis. You can cure this, but the cause of it was multifactorial, including your lifestyle choices and lack of self-care. Unless you make a decision to stop abusing your body, no matter what steps are taken now, your symptoms will come back—with a vengeance."

That got his attention. Josh stuck with the program.

We did have to talk more about thinking with all three of his brains. He hadn't really taken this seriously. He was still ignoring signals.

But at the 180-day follow-up, Josh had lost about thirty pounds. He looked more grounded and present, and he'd taken up coaching his daughter's soccer team. And he'd decided—after Anabel showed him cardiologist Dr. Dean Cornish's research on diet and cardiovascular disease—to eat vegetarian at least four days a week. His libido had significantly improved (which Anabel privately thanked me for), his marriage was "better than I can remember," and his bloating had decreased by about seventy percent.

"Yep, I drank the Kool-Aid, Doc," he laughed, "and it worked! I finally understand what you meant by connecting my three brains!"

Chronic Inflammation and Two of the Three Brains

A significant body of study in gastrointestinal function has shown that the combination of bloating, brain fog, headaches, anxiety, fatigue, and decreased cognition is caused by antibodies that compromise the blood-brain barrier. This leads to the leaking of toxins directly into the bloodstream, and that precipitates bloating. The allowance of harmful substances to cross directly into the system creates dangerous inflammatory conditions. Inflammation in the gut also significantly affects the production of neurotransmitters.

The magnitude of the critical functions of the gut is astounding. Ninety percent of serotonin, the happy hormone, is metabolized and stored in the gut. The gut is also home to neurotransmitters like dopamine, glutamate, norepinephrine, GABA (gamma-aminobutyric acid), and nitric oxide. Together, these neurotransmitters coordinate much of our vitality and well-being, including brain performance.

How the Three Brains Communicate with Each Other

The main highway for communication in our three brain connection is the vagus nerve. In Latin, vagus means "wandering."

It's the only cranial nerve that exits the skull and continues down, past your neck into the gut, servicing the brain-gut axis. A vital, key component of the Three Amigos connection, the vagus nerve links the enteric nervous system (ENS) to the brain. It also mediates lowering the heart rate.

Our Three Brains in Conflict

If you are like most people, you have probably experienced conflicts between your three brains. It usually feels something like this: The brain in your head points you in one direction, but your heart and/or gut say something else entirely. Or perhaps you've had that familiar, yet annoying sense that something is off, but when your brain looks for the "it" that's off, it finds nothing to concretely confirm your suspicion. Yet, you still feel like something's wrong. You may even think it's a figment of your hyperactive imagination. Health issues follow the same pattern and rapidly perpetuate if we fail to understand the connection between our three brains.

CASE STUDY

The Scared Kid and the Immigration Officer

I still remember it as if it were yesterday, even though it happened over 41 years ago. I was at the Miami airport, my first port of entry into the United States. I'd just turned nineteen. I had never been away from Brazil and was about to be interviewed by a not-so-friendly immigration officer. I could barely speak when he asked me, "What's the reason you're coming to the U.S.?"

Suddenly my hands were sweating profusely, my heart was pounding, and I felt a bit woozy in the head. I had a rush of butterflies in my stomach. My belly started hurting. I felt both bloated and nauseous. I had to go to the bathroom NOW, or I was afraid I was going to poop my pants.

The fight-or-flight response was in full force. My "gut" and "heart" brains wanted to flee—and my "head" brain had to come to the rescue.

I focused and, as calmly as I could, told him I was here to go to school, and he let me go. Literally.

Ever had something similar happen to you? This was an example of the significant and useful connection between the head, heart, and gut brains.

The Powerful Gut-Brain Axis

Our "three brains" clearly play a crucial role in preventing diseases and maintaining overall health. We have all experienced how the brain communicates with the gut. Phrases like "gut-wrenching" exemplify how our everyday communication utilizes our gut's feelings to denote our emotions. For some of us, specific situations can make us feel nauseous—or like we've been "punched in the gut." Expressions like this have come into common usage because gastrointestinal tract symptoms are often triggered by emotions such as anger, anxiety, sadness, or excitement.

In other words, the brain has a direct effect on the stomach and intestines. The very thought of eating, for example, releases the stomach's juices before the food even arrives. And this connection goes both ways. A troubled intestine sends signals to the brain, just as an anxious mind sends signals to the gut.

Because the Head Brain, Heart Brain, and Gut Brain are intimately connected, a person's stomach or intestinal distress (such as bloating) can grow worse due to anxiety, stress, or depression. Bloating affects our perception of ourselves (espe-cially when looking in the mirror), is often embarrassing, and may have no apparent physical cause. It's no surprise that anxi-ety and depression often are co-presenting factors.

Gastroenterologists and internists also know that patients with gastrointestinal problems often experience anxiety and stress due to their condition—and that anxiety and stress can, in turn, make the GI problems even worse. It can be a vicious spiral, with no end in sight.

The Heart-Brain Connection

The communication between the heart and brain is dynamic. Utilizing a two-way approach, each "brain" continuously influ-ences and supports the other's functions. Studies have shown that the heart and the brain utilize four different ways to communi-cate: *neurologically* (through the transmission of nerve impulses), *biochemically* (via hormones and neurotransmitters), *biophysically* (through pressure waves), and *energetically* (through electromag-netic field interactions).[1] Constant communication via these four mechanisms enhances brain activity and performance.

Most of us have experienced how the heart communicates with the brain and significantly affects how we perceive and react to the world. Our heart knows our brain well and knows that without a connection between the two of them, our world would be bland indeed.

In fact, more and more studies are showing us that when patients with gastrointestinal conditions have psychology-based approaches added to their treatments, they make significant improvements in their digestive symptoms (as compared to patients who received only conventional medical treatment). This is why an all-around treatment for bloating must also address the psychological impacts of this condition.

8

Metabolism, Blood Flow, Sex, and Hormones

"Hormone balance is the pearl of healthy metabolism—
and hence increased longevity."

—E. de Mello, MD, PhD

D erived from Greek, the word *hormone* means to excite or set in motion. Hormones are essential, and they can be a nightmare when they get out of balance.

Hormones are chemicals produced by glands in the endocrine system and are essential to all of the metabolic processes needed for our survival. They travel through the bloodstream delivering messages, signaling, and instructing the body on what to do. These messages range from simple alerts—like telling us that our body needs food or water—to reminding us to go to sleep or to wake up. These signals can stress us out, calm us down, or even get us aroused for sex. The vital role that hormones play in our everyday lives is like no other. Our bodies are regulated by hormones for our entire lives—from the moment we are conceived to our final breath.

Endocrinology is the field of study that explains how hormones work. One of the reasons we are able to live longer is because of our growing understanding of the essential role hormones play in our lives.

From pre-puberty, to adolescence, to middle and old age, the effects that hormones have on our bodies and minds are far-reaching. Most of us have, at one time or another, experienced how hormonal deficiencies can wreak total havoc on our immune and gastrointestinal systems, our libidos, cognition, and overall mental balance.

In addition to aiding in our digestion, hormone balance is also essential to longevity and healthy aging. Studies by John Morrison, an expert on the neurobiology of aging, have shown that estrogen is essential in restoring synaptic health and improving working memory. That is, age-related cognitive decline is now believed to be in part due to estrogen and testosterone deficiency.[1,2]

What Exactly Happens When Our Hormones Are Out of Whack?

When hormonal imbalances occur—that is, when there is too much or too little of them in the bloodstream—there can be devastating consequences for the body. Because hormones are vital for regulating most major bodily processes, even small imbalances can cause an array of troublesome symptoms. Hormonal imbalances can significantly decrease the function of most organ systems, including:

- Gastrointestinal system: bloating, irregular bowel movements, cramps, mood swings
- Reproductive cycles and sexual function: low libido, male erectile dysfunction, infertility
- Metabolism and appetite: overeating, under-eating, water retention, weight gain
- Mood and stress: anxiety, depression, irritability, suicidal ideation

- Body temperature: chills, hot flashes
- Heart rate: irregular heartbeat, heart fluttering, heart disease
- Sleep cycles: insomnia, oversleeping

We tend to think of estrogen as "female" and testosterone as "male," but all of us have both of these hormones. Many women have experienced the effects of estrogen and progesterone during their menstrual cycles when they become bloated. In men, a decrease in testosterone due to normal aging can be accompanied by an increase in levels of estrogen, and sometimes with distressing effects.

Hormonal Cycles: Male and Female

The female cycle has four phases: menstruation, follicular, ovulation, and luteal. The luteal phase begins soon after ovulation and lasts for two weeks. During this phase, the uterus's main job is to prepare for a possible pregnancy. Estrogen decreases significantly and then suddenly starts to increase again, creating the emotional roller coaster that some women experience.

Not all women suffer from it, but for those who do, bloating, mood swings, insomnia, depression, and overeating are among the most challenging results of this hormonal roller coaster.

If a pregnancy occurs, a woman's progesterone levels go up and stay up! If pregnancy does not occur, the uterine lining then sheds, and menstruation happens, restarting the whole cycle.

These hormonal swings can, of course, wreak havoc on the digestive tract. It has been described by many women as "Hormone Hell."

And then . . .

For women, eventually menopause happens, and the ovaries atrophy. That is, even when there is an attempt to signal the body to release an egg (ovum), there are no more eggs left to be released. Eventually, both estrogen and progesterone levels stay low, and the endometrium starts to atrophy.

Luteinizing hormone (LH) and follicle-stimulating hormone (FSH) are called *gonadotropins* because they stimulate the gonads: ovaries in females, the testes in males. The spike of FSH and LH during menopause causes well-documented menopausal symptoms: cramping, flushing, hot flashes, headaches, irritability, and—you guessed right—BLOATING!

How Estrogen and Progesterone Cause Women to BLOAT Like a Balloon

Progesterone levels are higher in the latter half of a woman's cycle, which in turn slows the digestive tract. Water and/or gas retention then ensues, usually in the midsection of the stomach, leading to bloating or an uncomfortable feeling of being "too full."

The water retention that most women experience during their period occurs mainly in this latter half of a woman's menstrual cycle. During this time, estrogen levels are also increased. Because estrogen causes women to retain water, this leads to further increased bloating. Post-menopausal women also bloat and retain water because their estrogen levels tend to increase and decrease irregularly.[3] Progesterone is a diuretic, which means it leads to more peeing. Decreased levels of this hormone will often contribute to water retention.[4] While painful water retention from hormone imbalances commonly occurs in the midsection, it can also occur outside of the stomach area in the feet, hands, and face.

Interestingly, in women, low levels of estrogen are linked to osteoporosis (when bones become less dense, weaker, and more brittle), but in men decreased levels of testosterone have been linked to osteoporosis. Tests find that men with lower testosterone levels often have less bone density, just like women with low estrogen do.

What About Dudes? Do We Have a Cycle?

Yes, we do!

In men, the equivalent of menopause is called *andropause.* Commonly known as "male menopause," the term refers to age-related changes in male hormone levels, leading to a group of symptoms, among them testosterone deficiency, androgen deficiency, and late-onset hypogonadism.

Testosterone is produced mainly by cells in the gonads in men (ovaries in women), with a small amount of testosterone produced in the adrenal glands of both sexes. You may have seen the ads, but the function of testosterone is more than just enhancing our sex drive! Testosterone also aids in our mental, physical, and emotional health, as well as increasing and strengthening muscle mass, regulating cortisol (and the fight-or-flight response), and giving men their more masculine features.

Andropause is associated with the loss of sexual potency, which in some men can bring on a crisis of confidence and identity. It's what's called a "midlife crisis."

Like women during menopause, during this time, men may experience symptoms such as:

- Reduced muscle mass
- Erectile dysfunction
- Low libido
- Gynecomastia (increased breast size)
- Feelings of physical weakness
- Low energy
- Lowered self-confidence
- Difficulty concentrating
- Depression or sadness

- Decreased motivation
- Insomnia
- Increased body fat

Where, in women, normal aging and menopause eventually lead to a complete shutdown in their reproductive organs, in men, the effects of andropause are often less obvious or pronounced. And although men's reproductive organs are not shut down, per se, men can still face sexual complications due to their decreased testosterone levels.

Swollen or tender breasts, decreased testicle size, loss of body hair—and yes, guys, even hot flashes—are some of the most common indicators of decreased testosterone levels in men.

When Does "Male Menopause" Happen?

Current research shows that after age thirty, testosterone levels in men tend to decline by an average of one percent each year. Certain medical conditions, such as obesity, extreme weight loss, metabolic syndrome (including high blood pressure or high cholesterol levels), or HIV/AIDS[5] can cause early and/or more drastic declines in testosterone levels.

Andropause lasts up to fifteen to twenty years in some men, while the body adjusts to increasingly low testosterone levels. Some men don't feel any strong effects of decreasing testosterone as they age. Lucky dudes!

But What Do Hormones Have to Do With My Gut Health?

The connection between the microbiome, gut health, and hormone utilization and balance is so strong that a term has been coined to denote this relationship. The *estrobolome* is the specific set of bacterial genes, the *code* for the enzymes that metabolize estrogen in our guts. What this means is that the gut flora can predispose anybody—woman or man—to have either too *much* estrogen or to have an estrogen/testosterone *deficiency* based on how certain species of bacteria in the gut are metabolizing estrogen. This leads to inflammatory conditions in the body and increased risk of some cancers.

Balanced hormones play an important role in the GI tract, digestion, and the immune system. Did you know that an estimated 70% of women experience bloating during their period? Men also experience bloating when they have hormonal imbalances.

Both men and women are affected by imbalances in hormone metabolism, which, in turn, have an effect on insulin, steroid hormones, and growth hormones. With all these changes comes the universal symptom of bloating.

In women, imbalances of the hormones estrogen and progesterone can heavily affect the speed of digestion. These imbalances can lead to symptoms like diarrhea, nausea, and abdominal pain when food is rushed through the system. Or if food moves too slowly, it can also cause bloating and constipation.

Post-menopausal women, in particular, commonly have to deal with adverse, hard-to-diagnose symptoms. Here's the problem: according to many of my female patients complaining of severe bloating and constipation, their doctors can never really nail down what's wrong with them. I find it astounding that more physicians don't make the connection with hormone imbalances when patients complain of bloating or constipation.

Estrogen levels also affect different organs in the GI tract, like the gallbladder. The role of the gallbladder is to release bile, which aids in digestion and the absorption of nutrients. When there are excess levels of estrogen, bile thickens, and this can sometimes lead to the creation of gallstones. Taking birth control pills, which provide extra amounts of estrogen, can also lead to this development.[6] However, if there is too little bile production due to decreased levels of estrogen, then digestion and absorption will slow, and stool will accumulate in excess.[7] This too can lead to painful and annoying bloating and constipation.

But sex hormones like progesterone and estrogen aren't the only types of hormones that affect the GI tract. A study by Nagisa Sugaya found that dehydroepiandrosterone (DHEA) and cortisol levels (both adrenal hormones involved in cell repair and healing of the immune system) have an effect on the symptoms for those with IBS.[8] The study found that people with IBS had lower levels of DHEA and higher levels of cortisol after an induced stressful event than did those without IBS.[9] This indicates that the stress of IBS symptoms can prolong the symptoms themselves because of how these hormones affect the immune system.

More About Hormones . . .

Thyroid hormones also disrupt digestive system functions. Individuals with hypothyroidism (low thyroid levels) can experience chronic constipation because their digestion slows down.

Melatonin, a hormone that is produced in the stomach during meals and in the brain during sleep, can help with bloating by regulating stomach acid. It also increases the production of an enzyme called *pepsin*, whose function is to move food from the stomach into the intestines.

Then there's that pesky *leptin*, the so-called "fat hormone." It is a protein hormone produced by fat cells. Leptin's main role is to tell your brain to use the body's fat stores for energy. One of the most common reasons some of my patients have a difficult time losing weight is due to what's called "leptin resistance," a type of hormonal imbalance that interrupts communication between the brain and the body's fat stores, making shedding those extra pounds difficult.

Tips and Treatments for Hormonal Imbalances

Although treatments for hormonal imbalances vary depending on factors like medical history, age, and ethnicity, there are common denominators. Here are a few tips on how you can better control your own hormonal balance to avoid bloating and other gastrointestinal issues. Some may already look familiar to you.

Tips:
- Eat a nutritious and balanced diet.
- Avoid fruits and vegetables that have been sprayed with pesticides or ripening chemicals.
- Exercise regularly.
- Maintain a healthy body weight.
- Reduce and manage stress.
- Practice yoga, meditation, or any other relaxation technique.
- Avoid sugary foods and refined carbohydrates.
- Avoid processed foods.
- Avoid microwaving foods and drinks, especially in plastic containers.
- Restrict the use of toxic cleaning products.

The Integrative Approach

Natural supplements to treat hormonal imbalances have been in existence since practically the beginning of time. Ancient cultures used the "natural approach" (think Chinese and Ayurvedic medicine). They have provided us with a rich approach to treating hormonal imbalance. But research in the natural approach to treat hormones has been scarce, largely due to "lack of interest" from the pharmaceutical industry. Currently, there are no extensive clinical studies proving the effectiveness of natural remedies for treating hormonal imbalances and their causes.

And why would they be interested? There's less money in it for pharmaceutical companies!

However, small, independent studies have shown the effectiveness of one approach over the other. It turns out that properly used plant medicines really can help. For example, black cohosh, dong quai, red clover, and evening primrose oil are all used to treat hot flashes and have been found to be some of the most effective herbs for optimizing and balancing hormones.

In addition, ginseng has been proven effective for irritability, anxiousness, and sleep disturbances in both men and women. Ginseng combined with maca, if taken while making lifestyle changes like getting more exercise, eating a healthy diet, and reducing stress, have been shown to be effective in treating men with erectile dysfunction. How about that!

CASE STUDY

"I just can't deal with this anymore."

Hannah was in her early fifties when she first came to see me. For the past ten years, she had been suffering from severe bloating and, as she described it, "Puffiness every-goddamn-where! I used to be in perfect health," she said.

"I worked like a woman possessed. I had two kids, got divorced, remarried, and then had another kid with my second husband. Then, by the time I was forty-five, it felt like all hell broke loose." She hesitated, then confessed, "Dr. de Mello, if I didn't have kids who need me, I think I would've taken myself out by now. I am often so swollen, *everywhere*! My face is puffy, and my stomach hurts all the time. I don't see even the slightest bit of my former self when I look in the mirror."

Hannah—who is actually a practicing oncologist—bit one side of her lip, and then squeaked out, "Help me, Doc!"

After spending two hours interviewing Hannah and assessing her history, it was clear to me that her previous practitioners had not considered the effects of having three kids over ten years on her body and her hormones. In my practice, it is vital we consider all possible causes. I started with evaluating her gut health.

As I have mentioned, the gut contributes to almost every chronic health problem. Hannah's hormone blood panel revealed that her estrogen levels were extremely high compared to her progesterone. Her stool test showed complete dysbiosis, and her thyroid levels revealed that she was slightly hypothyroid. The dysbiosis had left Hanna severely compromised with intestinal permeability. This created systemic inflammation, which set her gastrointestinal and endocrine systems spiraling out of control.

Hannah's hypothyroid needed to be tackled next. The hypothalamic-pituitary-adrenal (HPA) axis is extremely important when considering hormone imbalance issues. The hypothalamus and the pituitary glands regulate all hormone production in the body, including thyroid, adrenal, and sex hormones.

In Hannah's case, the cortisol and HPA axis dysfunction led to a "freezing" of her HPA. In other words, it was shell-shocked and unable to operate fully, causing Hannah to have a severe decrease in her energy, libido, and control of her emotions. In her own words: "I behaved like a crazy woman most of the time."

Hannah's cortisol levels were also off the charts. Cortisol is the stress response hormone that, at high levels, can cause hormone resistance, where receptors on cells become less sensitive and less able to activate the transceptors to have the proper reactions. Hannah's high cortisol levels led to insulin resistance, and her endocrine system had become unable to metabolize like it was supposed to.

In an insulin resistant person, the very cells that need insulin for metabolism have become insensitive to it, leading to what is referred to as insulin resistance or Metabolic Syndrome—the first step toward diabetes. This was one of the causes of Hannah's weight gain and malaise, as well as her edema (water retention) and bloating.

Hannah's treatment plan involved a multidisciplinary approach at Akasha Clinic. Her pelvic ultrasound revealed a very thin uterine lining, but no masses. This indicated that Hannah was a perfect candidate for the bio-identical hormone replacement (BIHRT). After her genetic testing and family history revealed no risk for breast cancer, she was placed on a bio-identical hormone.

Then, Hannah met with our integrative nutritionist and was placed on a low FODMAP diet. Under my care, she was treated using an integrative approach, combining both Eastern and Western remedies.

When I met with her for a six-month visit, Hannah looked like a different person. She beamed, "I have not felt this good in such a long time!" She had followed our suggestion and hired a trainer to come to her office, exercising at a nearby park three times a week. She had taken up a weekend yoga class when her husband could watch the kids, and she had embraced the infrared sauna like a savior. The sweating allowed her skin (the largest organ of the body) to detox, and she found it was relaxing.

After just one year of sticking to my treatment plan, Hannah says she has been feeling the absolute best she has felt in her adult life. She has a lot more energy, exercises consistently, and also spends more quality time with her children. She is not constantly stressed. She feels like herself again.

Due to her many previous failed visits to physicians who could not diagnose what was wrong with her body, Hannah was extremely impressed with our integrative approach to medicine. In fact, she was so impressed with the ability of this regimen to get to the root cause of symptoms that she decided to start a fellowship in integrative medicine. There is no doubt that Hannah will be able to save lives and ease stress once armed with integrative medical training!

CHAPTER 9

Treatment Approaches

"Without trust, there's no effective communication
and hence no viable relationship."

—E. de Mello, MD

Okay, so now we know about the many potential causes of bloating, and fortunately, there are just as many ways to treat it. Making a commitment to lifestyle changes paired with eating an appropriate diet and taking the right supplements or medications when necessary will put you well on your way towards a bloat-free tummy! In the following pages, you will find an outline and description of my treatment approach, along with information on nutrition, and natural and herbal treatments, plus essential questions to ask the practitioner treating your gas and bloating.

PART I: Treatment Guidelines

1. Be Open, and Trust Your Practitioner

As we've discussed, there are usually numerous contributing factors to increased gas and bloating. These include a slew of disorders, such as SIBO and IBS, and a number of pre-existing conditions, such as hormonal imbalances, that might have led to your bloated stomach. It is, therefore, vitally important to be specific about the details of your symptoms when you speak to your doctor. Be ready to share any potential triggers you have noticed. Have you noticed what makes the bloating better or worse? What has and what has not worked in the past to relieve your symptoms?

I believe that any treatment protocol should be based on an effective and trusting physician-patient relationship combined with an integrative and behavioral approach. To evaluate the symptoms, and hopefully eradicate the conditions, a trusting therapeutic relationship must be fostered. When this happens, the patient feels "seen" and the healing process starts even before a plan is fully implemented.

The truth is, there is no standardized, one-size-fits-all, evidence-based protocol for treating patients with bloating issues. A comprehensive, personalized, integrative treatment plan must be developed for each individual patient. For example, are you bloated or distended or both? Identifying your chief symptoms is always the first step because it can provide valuable insights to the underlying root cause of the problem.

2. Ask the Right Questions

Before we get into the specifics on how to improve your bloating problem, you should know that you should never be afraid to assert yourself with your doctor. Ask any questions about your body that concern you.

"Why does my body bloat even after I eat *a salad* filled with nutritious vegetables or regardless of *what* I eat?"

Maybe you need to ask, "Why does it hurt when I use the bathroom?"

These are all good questions if you have them on your mind.

When your doctor is explaining your treatment plan with you, you should make sure you completely understand. Always ask about anything they say that is not clear to you. After all, this is valuable information that is supposed to benefit your body, and it does no good if you don't understand what the heck your doctor is talking about.

3. Educate Yourself

What is your bloated body trying to tell you? Your body talks to you by using its own unique language—through your *symptoms*. Something feels wrong, and the body communicates that information to you. Then you talk to your doctor, and the practitioner has to interpret the body's language. You need to be as clear as possible in describing what is going on with you.

Together, you and your doctor can come up with an effective and relatively easy-to-follow regimen. Specific and reasonable goals are identified, and a roadmap is developed for how each issue will be tackled.

For example, I educate my patients that every day, adults produce one to three pints of gas on average. This gas is passed through the anus. Some might believe that producing so much gas must be an indication they are unhealthy. It isn't. I have to emphasize the fact that passing some gas is not only normal; it is *healthy*.

Some people lack the enzymes they need to digest certain carbohydrates, including starch, sugar, fiber, and others found in a wide variety of foods. Bloating occurs when the undigested carbohydrates travel from the small intestine, undigested, into the large intestine, where they have to be broken down by gas-producing bacteria. One of the gases these bacteria produce is *sulfur*, which, as you know, is not known for its sweet-smelling properties.

4. Watch Your Diet

If there is a universal "first step" for anyone with a health problem like bloating, it is to look at (and change) their DIET. In other words, you really should not expect your human machine to perform at a very high level if you are fueling it with processed junk. That is why I take time to thoroughly interview each of my patients as to their dietary history and habits.

I am especially interested in their consumption of food products that can readily ferment in the colon—dairy, fructose, fructans, fiber, and sorbitol. I inform my patients about sugars with the highest potential to cause gas. Some foods contain more than one of these culprits.

I tell them to (initially) avoid beans, cabbage, brussels sprouts, broccoli and other cruciferous_vegetables, and whole grains.

Finally, I explain that the enzyme lactose, contained in milk products such as ice cream and cheese, is also a component of processed foods, including cereal and salad dressings, and should be initially avoided.

Befriend an Anti-Inflammation Diet

As previously addressed, inflammation is the biggest challenge that every organ system faces daily, making it the number one underlying cause behind most diseases and imbalances. Given that inflammation and toxicity are common denominators in so many maladies, the primary goal of a dietary program is to eliminate inflammation, while at the same time seeking to discover why the patient's GI system is not operating optimally.

Contributors to chronic inflammation include:

- **Fried foods:** cooked with trans fats and vegetable oils
- **Factory farmed meats**
- **Highly processed/packaged foods**
- **Refined carbohydrates** like grains, sugars, alcohol
- **Artificial food additives**
- **Dairy**
- **Environmental toxins:** pesticides/herbicides, dust,

mold, harmful chemicals and so many "personal care" products
* **Allergies and food intolerances**
* **Stress and toxic emotions:** unhealthy relationships, negative thoughts/feelings

All of these can cause overgrown or unbalanced gut bacteria, leading to small intestinal bacterial overgrowth (SIBO), inflammatory bowel disease (IBD) and other syndromes that negatively affect your gut.

You can find a more extensive list and explanation of FOD-MAPS in Chapter 5: Nutrition.

Be Aware of "Die-off"

Also known as the *Herxheimer reaction*, die-off occurs as the result of a sudden increase in endotoxins (or bacterial waste) when bacteria and other microbes die. When this happens, your immune system creates an immune response that can lead to a temporary worsening of the very symptoms that led you to take the remedy in the first place.

Although die-off is also known as a possible reaction to antifungals or antibiotics, a change in a diet—like a detox or cleanse—can also lead to die-off and its accompanying symptoms. Remember that the bacteria and yeast that live in our gut thrive on sugar. Some of these microorganisms are essential for proper digestion, elimination, and even detoxing our digestive system. However, a diet high in carbs, sugar, and alcohol significantly increases the number of these organisms, overwhelming the immune system.

Some people even feel like they are drunk during die-off. This is because of the metabolites released when certain cells are destroyed. For example, when Candida cells die, they release acetaldehyde, a by-product produced when we consume alcohol.

Bloating, nausea, headaches, brain fog, abdominal discomfort, and sometimes vomiting are also symptoms of die-off. It usually lasts three to seven days.

Easing the Side Effects

Slow down. Be gentle on yourself. Support your body's innate detox mechanism. Remember, there is no need to rush. You are not in competition with your harmful bacteria. You are stronger than they are! Move slowly and gently into a diet with fewer sugars and carbs.

5. Consider Supplements

There are several supplements that can naturally help your system defend itself against the overgrowth of bacteria, yeast, and other microorganisms. Some of the best supplements to take during die-off include:

- **Glutathione:** Considered a *scavenger antioxidant amino acid* as well as an immunity booster, glutathione is undoubtedly among the best and most potent cleansers and detoxifiers.
- **Vitamin C**, 2,000–3000 mg mgs a day, and **N-acetyl Cysteine (NAC)**, 1,800 mg a day. Both of these minimize the oxidative damage caused by the die-off toxins.
- **Coconut Charcoal:** One capsule in the morning and one capsule in the evening helps flush toxins from your body safely by binding to the harmful toxins.
- **Eat Your Veggies:** beets, radishes, artichokes, cabbage, broccoli, spirulina, chlorella, and seaweed help to cleanse us and alleviate the symptoms of die-off by supporting the liver's detoxification.

o **Dandelion root**, **burdock**, and **milk thistle** are herbs that have been shown to help both detox and die-off.

o In addition, drinking **green tea** and adding a mixture of organic greens to your diet that contain the chelators **spirulina and chlorella** (such as *Akasha Naturals Vital Greens*) can significantly help boost the immune system. Take these at least three times a week in the morning, and add the greens mixture to your water in the evening before bed three times a week.

o **Digestive Enzymes:** Taking two digestive enzyme capsules before meals, such as *Akasha Naturals' Digestazyme*, can enhance digestion and improve elimination. As a sidenote, do not use fungal or plant-based enzymes as they will likely make the symptoms worse.

Beyond Supplements . . .

• **Extra Virgin Olive Oil:** Add 1–2 tablespoons to your food twice a day. Or even more effective, take it on an empty stomach, at least 4 hours away from food.

• **Flaxseed** and **Chia Seed**: Help firm up your stool for easier elimination. Mix two tablespoons into water, stir, and allow the mixture to sit for ten minutes. Like olive oil, it is best on an empty stomach.

• **Water:** Drink plenty of it. Water increases the elimination of toxins by strengthening your detoxification through urine. I recommend drinking half of your body weight in ounces. For example, if you weigh 120 pounds, you need to drink 60 ounces per day.

• **Sweating:** Don't forget that sweating is a good way to detox! Sweat via exercise or sauna (infrared is best), at least three times a week.

- **Oatmeal baths** have been shown to soothe itching and rashes. Soak for 30–45 minutes.
- **Get PLENTY of zzzz:** Sleep is rejuvenation for your body. The detox mechanisms or pathways are the most active when you are asleep.
- **Poop at least once a day:** Your body will absorb the toxins released during die-off if you do not have a bowel movement every day. **Magnesium Citrate** can help.
- **Stop dairy consumption!**

Evolutionarily speaking, dairy is not necessary for the optimal health of humans. Different cultures around the world have consumed dairy for thousands of years. Studies have documented that human genes have changed to accommodate dairy products in the diet.[1]

But *one does not need dairy* to fulfill the daily protein or calcium requirements. There are a variety of protein and calcium sources that will easily meet these requirements. The truth is that dairy consumption is actually unnatural for humans. Vegan children, and even animals such as gorillas and chimpanzees, do not drink milk or eat other protein from other animals. They do just fine eating plant-based proteins.

A 2012 study reported that approximately 75% of the world's population loses the ability to digest dairy at some point in their lives.[2] What I have seen in my practice is that a significant number of people with bloating problems are lactose intolerant.

The best (free) test you can do is to stop consuming dairy products and see how your body responds. Read the labels and eliminate any foods in which dairy is listed among the ingredients.

6. Add a Consistent Exercise Plan Emphasizing Posture

Exercise has been proven over and over again to help relieve stress, decrease pain, and even decrease the symptoms of depression and anxiety—especially when practiced consistently. Staying active improves elimination by increasing circulation. Exercise also optimizes the movement of lymphatic fluid throughout the body, helping the body to detox.

As discussed earlier, we all have experienced how connected the gut is to our body and brain. So just about anything that we can do to relieve stress will likely help with bloating. However, because gas retention is worse in the supine position (lying down) than upright, I advise my patients to exercise in an upright position, such as on a stationary bike. But don't overdo it! Too much straining puts the body into a stressful state where adrenal glands release a higher amount of cortisol, the so-called "stress hormone." Too many sit-ups, for example, can also overstrain your abdominal muscles and cause more bloating. The secret is to make sure your exercise regimen is well planned. Consult with a trainer at your gym or a physical therapist. If you exercise at home, seek out the right regimen, designed specifically for you.

7. Find Relaxation Techniques to Reduce Stress

We live in a world where we are bombarded daily with negative news. Stress is inevitable. When we are anxious or sad, this vital and complex line of communication is significantly affected.

A regular practice of deep relaxation has rich health benefits, including alleviating bloating symptoms.

When stress is not managed well, it can imprison us in a cycle of ongoing fight-or-flight response. This never-ceasing stress is detrimental to our physical, emotional, and spiritual wellness. It is as if we've jumped on a treadmill but cannot get off.

Faced with the challenges of this fight-or-flight response, the brain turns on its survival mode and diverts attention away from proper digestion and elimination in order to conserve the energy needed to survive. Personally, I do not know how some people manage to live our busy and often demanding modern lives without a daily relaxation technique. Without mine, I'd go completely bonkers, cuckoo, kaput!

My Prescription

Start by making your mealtime *"me* time." Practice mindful eating. Be aware of what you're putting in your body. Be grateful that you have food to sustain your body. Put your fork down between bites. Taste. Chew. Nourish.

And whether you have ten minutes or one hour, make relaxation a part of your daily protocol. Treat yourself, decreasing stress with meditation (or the technique of your choice). Taking this time for yourself will help to lessen your bothersome symptoms and will ultimately heal you.

PART II: Medications

1. Over the Counter (OTC) Laxatives Vs. Natural Laxatives

Because laxatives can cause electrolyte imbalances, their use can lead to serious side effects. Like many OTC drugs, some laxatives can actually make your bloating symptoms worse. In addition, the overuse of laxatives decreases bowel function, eventually making one's system dependent on them. Additionally, laxatives should NEVER be used for weight loss! If absolutely needed, use them cautiously and only under a doctor's supervision.

Instead of commercial laxatives, I usually recommend foods that are known to be natural laxatives:

Chia Seeds: rich in natural fiber, which for some is the first line of defense against the constipation that can accompany bloating. Increasing fiber intake can increase stool frequency, soften stools, and ease their passage. Chia seeds move through the intestines undigested, adding bulk and encouraging regularity.

Berries: High in fiber, berries are both a mild natural laxative and antioxidant. Berries contain both soluble and insoluble fibers. Soluble fiber absorbs water in the gut to form a gel-like substance that helps soften stool (like with chia seeds). Insoluble fiber does not absorb water but moves through the body intact, increasing the bulk of stool for easier elimination.

Flaxseeds: high in omega-3 fatty acid and protein. Flaxseeds are also rich in nutrients making them a healthy food that also has natural laxative properties. Flaxseeds contain a mix of soluble and insoluble fiber. I recommend using one tablespoon (10 grams) of flaxseeds (which provides 2 grams of insoluble fiber and 1 gram of soluble fiber) once or twice a day to alleviate constipation.

Legumes: Belonging to a family of foods that include beans, chickpeas, lentils, green peas and peanuts, legumes are rich in fiber. One cup of boiled lentils, for example, contains 15.6 grams of fiber, while 1 cup of chickpeas provides 12.5 grams of fiber. Legumes are also known to increase the production of *butyric acid*, a type of short-chain fatty acid that acts as a natural laxative. Butyric acid is an anti-inflammatory agent, reducing intestinal inflammation.

Magnesium Citrate: a scientifically proven effective laxative. Magnesium citrate is better absorbed in the body than other forms of magnesium. It facilitates bowel movements by increasing the amount of water in the intestinal tract.

Castor Oil: produced from castor beans. Castor oil has a long history of use as a natural laxative. It is rich in *ricinoleic acid*, an unsaturated fatty acid known to reduce straining, soften the stool and decrease the sensation of incomplete evacuation.

Leafy Greens: nutrient-dense with vitamins, minerals and fiber and low in calories. Leafy greens such as kale and cabbage improve regularity and prevent constipation. The high level of magnesium (a proven laxative) present in these greens works by drawing more water into the intestines to facilitate elimination.

Senna: commonly found in popular over-the-counter laxatives such as Senokot, Senna Lax, and Ex-Lax. Senna leaf, scientifically known as *Senna alexandrina,* has been popular in the form of tea or powder for centuries, and dates back to two Arab physicians in the ninth century. Senna can be present in high amounts in rhubarb teas. Although proven effective, Senna has some side effects. It can make bloating worse and can sometimes cause stomach cramps and flu-like symptoms. It can become dangerous to your system if you take it long term.

Note: The proper dosage of Senna has not been standardized. Patients dealing with any liver, kidney, heart, Crohn's diseases, or other digestive system dysfunction should discuss the use of Senna with a knowledgeable practitioner. Women who are attempting to get pregnant or are pregnant or breastfeeding now should not take Senna without prior medical advice.

Apples are rich in pectin, a soluble fiber. Apples increase the level of beneficial bacteria in the gut, promoting better digestion, and functioning as a prebiotic. Apples speed up transit time in the colon, thereby improving elimination.

Kiwi is also rich in pectin as well as fiber. A 2007 study looked at the effects of kiwifruit on both constipated and healthy Chinese subjects. It found that kiwi increases the movement of the digestive tract to stimulate bowel movements, proving that it works as a natural laxative by speeding up transit time in the gut.[3]

Olive Oil functions as a lubricant by forming a coating in the rectum that promotes the easier passage of stool while also stimulating the small intestine to speed up transit.

Aloe Vera contains compounds that stimulate the movement of the digestive tract, alleviating constipation by drawing water into the intestines.[4]

Oat Bran is high in both soluble and insoluble fiber, making it an effective choice for a natural laxative. One cup of oat bran packs fourteen grams of fiber. In a geriatric hospital in 2009, a study designed to evaluate the effectiveness of oat bran to treat constipation instead of laxatives in a geriatric hospital in 2009 found it to be very effective.[5] The study's participants maintained their body weight, and 59% were able to stop using laxatives, proving that oat bran was a good alternative to over-the-counter laxatives.

Prunes are one of the most well-known natural laxatives in existence. Prunes contain a high amount of fiber: about two grams in each one-ounce serving. They also contain sorbitol, a type of sugar alcohol. Because sorbitol is poorly absorbed by the intestines, it acts as an osmotic agent, bringing water into the intestines and inducing bowel movements. Prunes can increase stool frequency and improve consistency better than many other natural laxatives.[6]

Coffee: Recent scientific studies on how coffee influences bowel habits are lacking, with most studies dating back to the 1990s. But coffee is known to stimulate the colon muscles, thereby producing a natural laxative effect for some individuals. The impact of coffee on elimination is mostly due to the fact that drinking it stimulates our production of *gastrin*, a hormone responsible for breaking down food in the stomach and pushing it through to be digested. In addition, the coffee bean contains phytonutrients and polyphenols, chemicals known to have antioxidant benefits. However, drinking more than two to three eight-ounce cups a day can cause insomnia and spikes in blood pressure and heart rate.

2. To Drink or Not to Drink?

Start by saying goodbye to drinks that are loaded with junk and artificial flavors; especially sugary, carbonated drinks! Sugary or carbonated beverages not only create bloating, but they are like a venom that quickly makes existing bloating problems even more uncomfortable.

Next is *alcohol*. It can kill the good bacteria in your gut while also suppressing your immune system. It can also make you bloat like a balloon.

I recommend drinking good ol' plain water! If you need to break the monotony of drinking water, I recommend adding slices of fresh fruit such as lemon or lime slices. Herbal teas like chamomile are also a good choice.

3. Probiotics and Prebiotics

Live microorganisms foster numerous health benefits. Probiotics have been found to help improve abdominal pain and discomfort, constipation, diarrhea, bloating, and other common bowel disorders. Having an unbalanced gut flora has been linked to numerous diseases, including obesity, type two diabetes, metabolic syndrome, heart disease, Alzheimer's, and depression.[7,8] Both probiotics and prebiotic fibers strengthen the function of our microbiota by helping correct this imbalance.[9] When starting a probiotic regimen, less is more. In other words, start low and slow. It is possible to experience some gas and bloating when starting a new probiotic supplement. It's always important to consult with a knowledgeable healthcare practitioner before starting.

What About Apple Cider Vinegar?

While apple cider vinegar has its perks, don't depend on it as your main or only source of probiotics. Consume a variety of probiotics found in fermented foods like yogurt, kefir, kimchi, sauerkraut, miso, tempeh, and kombucha tea.

4. Prescription Medications

In a study published in 2006 by the *American Journal of Gastro-enterology*, researchers reported for the first time that rifaximin, an antibiotic used to treat diarrhea, was an effective treatment for abdominal bloating and flatulence, including irritable bowel syndrome (IBS). The study conducted at the American University of Beirut in Lebanon found that rifaximin was effective in relieving the symptoms of bloating and excess gaseousness by way of reducing the amount of hydrogen gas produced in the large intestine. And because rifaximin is non-absorbable, there were no reported side effects. Rifaximin is a gut selective antibiotic that *is not* systemically absorbed and has little to no reported side effects.[10] Patients who are treated with rifaximin report improvement in bloating symptoms compared to patients who received placebo.[11]

PART III: Herbal Remedies and Treatments

Berberine: a compound found in several plants such as goldenseal, barberry, Oregon Grape, and tree turmeric. Berberine possesses multiple mechanisms that overcome bacterial resistance. It inhibits biofilm formation and reduces the number of hydrogen (H_2) producing bacteria, one of the main gases that cause bloating. Berberine has been a part of Chinese and Ayurvedic medicine for thousands of years. Although berberine appears to be safe, I recommend its use only under medical supervision given that it can cause nausea and, in some patients, make the bloating worse. Always consult a doctor before taking it.

Dose: 2–3 grams/day

Wormwood (*artemisia absinthium*): a green herb that makes a bitter tea. Wormwood can prevent or relieve indigestion by promoting the release of digestive juices that optimize digestion and decrease bloating. Wormwood also kills parasites, another culprit in bloating.[12]

Dose: One teaspoon (1.5 grams) of the dried herb per cup (about 250 ml) of boiling water. Steep it for five minutes and drink it slowly. The bitter taste can be softened by adding three to five drops of lemon juice and a teaspoon of raw honey. *Wormwood is inadvisable during pregnancy* because it contains *thujone*, a compound known to cause uterine contractions.

Ginger (*zingiber officinale*) has been used since ancient times for GI-related conditions, such as nausea.[13] Ginger speeds up stomach emptying after eating, thereby relieving bloating, gas, upset stomach, and intestinal cramping.

Dose: Take ginger capsules (1–1.5 grams) daily in two to three divided doses. For tea, add a half teaspoon (0.5–1.0 grams) of powdered, dried ginger root, or one tea bag per cup (250 ml) of boiling water. Steep for five minutes. Or you can use one tablespoon of fresh, sliced ginger in a boiling cup of water, and steep for ten minutes. Strain it and enjoy. Its spicy flavor can also be softened with honey and lemon.

Fennel seeds (*foeniculum vulgare*) are traditionally used to relieve bloating, gas, and other digestive disorders.[14] Similar in taste to licorice, fennel is also used to treat constipation, another contributing factor to bloating, because it is known to relieve sluggish bowels. Studies cite that when nursing-home residents suffering from chronic constipation drank one daily serving of an herbal tea with fennel seeds[15] their symptoms were relieved.

Dose: Add one or two teaspoons of seeds to a cup (250 ml) of boiling water. Steep for ten to fifteen minutes.

Gentian root (*Gentiana lutea*) is used as medicine for digestive issues such as stimulating appetite, curbing diarrhea, easing heartburn, and of course, bloating. It can also be applied to the skin to treat wounds and cancer.[16]

Dose: Add a half teaspoon of dried gentian root to a cup of boiling water. Steep for ten minutes. The tea may initially taste sweet, but a bitter taste follows. Some people prefer it mixed with chamomile tea and honey.

Chamomile (*Chamomillae romanae*) is used to treat bloating, gas, diarrhea, nausea, vomiting, and ulcers.[17] For centuries, chamomile has been effective in preventing *Helicobacter pylori*, a bacteria known for causing stomach ulcers and bloating.[18] Chamomile is also used to decrease abdominal pain and ulcers.[19] Its flowers contain one of the most beneficial flavonoids.

Dose: For tea, add one tablespoon of dried chamomile or one bag of chamomile tea to one cup of boiling water. Steep for ten minutes.

Angelica root (*Angelica archangelica*) is a member of the celery family. Angelica root extract stimulates digestive juices to promote healthy digestion[20] and prevent constipation, another culprit in bloating.

Dose: Add one teaspoon of the dried root to a cup of boiling water. Steep for five minutes. Given its bitter taste, steep it with lemon balm tea. Caution: because there is not enough information on its safety during pregnancy and breastfeeding, this herb should not be used under these conditions.

Caraway seeds: Caraway seeds have long been used to ease digestive gas and bloating due to its antispasmodic, antimicrobial and carminative effects. Caraway seeds help soothe the smooth muscle tissues of the digestive tract to release gas.

Dose: For frequent bloating, chew a few seeds several times throughout the day. Use caraway crackers instead if the taste

of raw caraway seeds is too strong. You can also brew crushed
caraway seeds to make tea.

Turmeric: Touted as one of the most powerful natural anti-
inflammatories, turmeric helps ensure the smooth functioning
of the digestive system. Curcumin, the active ingredient in turmeric, has been proven to reduce the symptoms of bloating and
gas. It facilitates the elimination of toxins in the feces while also
helping stimulate the gallbladder to produce bile to optimize
digestion and the absorption of fats and fat-soluble vitamins in
the small intestine.
Dose: Take one capsule before a meal or as a tea. It can be
added fresh or in powder form to foods and sauces. Or make
Golden Milk, a mixture of turmeric, almond or coconut milk,
cinnamon and honey to maximize the digestive benefits of turmeric. Mix one tsp. of turmeric powder, half a tsp. of cinnamon
powder and two tbsp. of honey into one cup of almond or coconut milk. Place the mixture in a pan and heat it until it's about
to boil. Make sure to cool the liquid a little before drinking it.

Cumin is an anti-inflammatory antioxidant with powerful antibacterial and antiseptic properties. Cumin seeds help get rid of
gas, strengthen the digestive tract, and relieve common bloating,
nausea, and constipation. Black cumin seeds offer a significantly
higher concentration of the medicinal cumin oil than the more
commonly available brown seeds.[21]
Dose: Combine a pinch of ground cumin, a pinch of sea salt,
and ground ginger in one cup of water. Drink twice a day, in the
morning and before bed.

Cinnamon: soothes the stomach and prevents further gas
buildup.
Dose: Add half a teaspoon of ground cinnamon to one cup of
warm water, almond or oat milk. Stir it well, and drink. You can

also add honey. Or add half a teaspoon of cinnamon powder (or a few cinnamon sticks) to one cup of boiling water. Steep for five minutes, and drink it twice a day.

Garlic: A member of the FODMAP "prohibited foods," the use of garlic to treat bloating has been somewhat controversial. It reduces the number of bacteria that produce methane (CH4), one of two common gases produced by gas-forming bacteria. Some people feel it helps with their bloating while others say this powerful natural antibiotic makes their bloating worse. Garlic's action against the overgrowth of yeasts in the gut makes it one of my choices for treating bloating in people who can tolerate it.
Dose: Try one 200 mg capsule three times a day. To both optimize digestion and extra flavor, mix minced raw garlic into your food.

Oregano (*oregano vulgare*) is a staple herb in cuisines around the world. The oil of oregano has been proven effective in reducing inflammation. In addition, oregano contains important nutrients. For example, one teaspoon of dried oregano contains 8% of the recommended daily amount of vitamin K.[22]
Dose: oil of oregano capsules (50-100 mg) twice a day. Start with the smaller dosage, 50 mg, and slowly increase to 100 mg twice a day.

Clove (*syzygium aromaticum*): Used for centuries in different cuisines, especially as one of the primary ingredients in Indian curries, clove is widely used in Ayurveda and traditional Chinese medicine as a pain reliever. Its antibacterial and antifungal properties are due to its high *eugenol* content, a natural antioxidant that helps fight inflammation by stimulating gastric mucus production. One teaspoon of cloves contains an impressive one gram of fiber,[23] plus manganese, a mineral that helps regulate blood sugar levels. It contains vitamin C that helps strengthen the immune system and vitamin K that helps regulate blood clotting.[24,25,26] A rinse mixed from clove, basil, and tea tree oil will significantly decrease the amount of plaque and bacteria in the mouth.

Dose: Add one teaspoon of ground cloves to your morning smoothie. Or simmer whole cloves in boiling water for five to ten minutes to make a soothing cup of clove tea.

Side effects: I do not recommend clove oil for children or for pregnant or breastfeeding women. Clove oil may cause seizures in children, liver damage, or fluid imbalances. Because the oil contains eugenol, which is known to decrease blood clotting, it should be avoided for at least two weeks before surgery.

Pomegranate (*punica granatum*): Food-borne diseases and those due to multi-drug resistant pathogens are now globally recognized as environmental hazards to our health and food supply. Pomegranates contain an impressive number of free-radical-fighting compounds that have strong antimicrobial properties. Extracts of pomegranate also contain phenolics and flavonoids which are potent inhibitors of several disease-causing bacteria. The value of pomegranate in bloating is due to its ability to combat some types of bacteria and the yeast, Candida albicans. This antimicrobial property gives pomegranates the ability to help prevent infection and antibiotic-resistant organisms, such as Methicillin-resistant Staphylococcus Aureus (MRSA). In addition, pomegranate contains two potent antioxidants, *punicalagins* and *punicic acid*, which have three times the antioxidant activity of red wine and green tea.[27,28]

Dose: I recommend using pomegranate juice because it readily enters the GI system to treat bloating and dyspepsia (heartburn). Drink 50–200ml of the juice daily or take powdered capsules. Or if you prefer the concentrated tincture, use 10 ml. daily of 1:2 tincture.

Uva Ursi (*arctostaphylos uva ursi*): Uva ursi means "bear's grape" in Latin, likely because bears love the fruit. First documented in the thirteenth century, this plant has been used in the treatment of urinary tract infections for centuries, but it also has well-known laxative properties. It was a common treatment for bladder infections until sulfa drugs and antibiotics were discovered. *Glycoside*, a chemical component of the herb, is converted into the powerful antibiotic-like compound *hydroquinone*, which reduces pathogenic bacteria causing constipation and bloating.

Uva Ursi's ability to fight infection comes from several chemicals, including *tannins* that tighten mucous membranes in the body. But be careful—it can also cause serious liver damage, if not taken properly.

Dose: Only the leaves, not the berries, are used in medicine. Use up to 10g of leaf daily. But start slowly and under the supervision of your doctor or an integrative practitioner.

Side effects: usually mild and include nausea and vomiting, irritability, and insomnia. Given its oxytocic properties (it stimulates the uterus), pregnant or breastfeeding women, as well as individuals with high blood pressure, Crohn's disease, digestive problems, kidney or liver disease, or ulcers should not take Uva Ursi. As with any herb, always discuss its use with your integrative practitioner as side effects and unwanted herbal/drug combinations can be dangerous.

Effectiveness: The preparation of Uva Ursi tends to be more effective when combined with green tea.

Pau d'arco (*tabebuia avellanedae*): Because it contains antimicrobial properties, more specifically anti-Candida, as early as 1873, pau d'arco has been used to kill bacteria, fungi, viruses, and parasites. It contains two chemicals, lapachol and beta-lapachone, which have been used to treat a wide range of inflammatory conditions, including the bloating that results from gastritis, gas pain, ulcers, liver conditions, diarrhea and nausea.

Dose: Not advised for children and infants. Adults: large amounts of pau d'arco can be toxic. It is best to find a standardized formula and do not take more than 1 gram a day.

Thyme (*thymus vulgaris*): Another Mediterranean import frequently used in the kitchen, thyme oil and its key constituent, *thymol*, are known for their antioxidant and muscle soothing activities, as well as their comfort for the stomach and relieving gas. Thyme oil supports a healthy balance of microflora in the gastrointestinal tract.

Rosemary (*rosmarinus officinalis*): While originating in the Mediterranean, it is now cultivated almost everywhere, including many kitchen herb gardens in the United States. Like peppermint, the essential oil of rosemary is well known for its ability to soothe digestive complaints and ease occasional abdominal discomfort by relaxing the muscles in the digestive tract. Rosemary stimulates appetite and improves gastric tone, allowing food to be eliminated more easily. (An interesting side note about rosemary is that due to its reputation for enhancing memory, rosemary has historically been referred to as a "symbol of remembrance," still sometimes carried or worn at Mediterranean weddings as a sign of loyalty and happiness.)

Black Walnut Hull (*Juglans nigra*): Used as a tonic to treat digestive issues, black walnut helps relieve heartburn, gas, and bloating. It stimulates the flow of bile into the intestines and is thought to ease abdominal pain. However, black walnut's most well-known property is its ability to fight intestinal parasites. This is due to its laxative properties that expel parasites, such as pinworm, ringworm, and tapeworm. Its high tannin and juglone content is believed to oxygenate the blood, thus helping to lower blood pressure and serum cholesterol levels. Due to its antifungal properties, black walnut has also been used to treat warts, herpes, cold sores, athlete's foot, and Candida.

Dose: Black walnut is extremely potent and should be used under the care of an integrative practitioner. Follow the suggested dose carefully. Use for no more than seven days in a row.

Peppermint (*Mentha piperita*) is recognized for helping to soothe digestive issues. The plant compound called flavonoids, found in a variety of plants, including peppermint, inhibits the activity of mast cells. Abundant in the gut, mast cells are a major component of the immune system that is known to contribute to bloating.[29]

Peppermint works by relaxing muscles, thus relieving bloating and intestinal spasms. Peppermint is also a natural pain reliever. Peppermint tea has been shown to be very potent, especially when steeped for a long time.

Dose: For tea, add either one tablespoon (1.5 grams) of dried peppermint leaves, one tea bag, or three tablespoons (17 grams) of fresh peppermint leaves to one cup (about 250 ml) of boiling water. Steep for ten minutes, strain it, and voila . . . your natural homemade bloating medicine is ready.

Lemon balm (*melissa officinali*): Lemon balm tea has been used to relieve bloating and other mild digestive issues. This lemon-scented herb, which is native to southern Europe, has historically been used as an anti-gas, antibacterial, and antispasmodic (to decrease cramps), and it has other non-GI related benefits, such as a memory-enhancing and tranquilizing agent.

Dose: Steep one tablespoon (3 grams) of dried lemon balm leaves, or one tea bag in one cup (250 ml) of boiling water for ten minutes.

Carminatives are known as an effective spasmolytic and for removing gas from the GI tract.

Examples of carminatives include caraway seeds, fennel, and anise.

Dose: A concoction for tea—crush together one tsp. of each caraway, fennel, and anise seeds. Steep the mixture for twenty minutes in one cup of water. Drink after each meal.

CAUTION: I list these herbs to educate, but keep in mind that self-prescribing herbs and other treatments can be dangerous. No one should take *all* of these herbs. It is essential that you consult with an integrative practitioner before starting any herbal regimen.

There are a variety of formulas in the market containing these herbs. Should you be interested in using herbs as a trial for the treatment of bloating, I strongly recommend working with an herbalist to make sure the herbs are of the highest quality and the dosage is accurate for you.

Do not self-diagnose, and do not self-prescribe. Always consult a licensed healthcare professional before you ingest herbs.

An Antibiotic-Like, Herbal Protocol for SIBO?

It was 2014, and one of those rare moments when a mainstream scholarly journal published a paper that addressed the effectiveness of herbal therapy over prescribed pharmaceutical antibiotics. It revolutionized the field of gastroenterology.

The study was called "Herbal Therapy Is Equivalent to Rifaximin for the Treatment of Small Intestinal Bacterial Overgrowth," and it was published in the *Journal of Global Advances in Health and Medicine*. One reason it was so impactful is that six of the study's nine authors were from the Johns Hopkins University Department of Gastroenterology.[30] Johns Hopkins is among the nation's top medical institutions.

I have dubbed this protocol "The Johns Hopkins Protocol" to emphasize to my patients the fact that a major Ivy League medical school agrees with what I have been doing for almost two decades. I treat bloating first with herbs and simple lifestyle changes—such as a healthy diet, good sleep, and exercise. I use antibiotics only if everything else has failed. Why? Because antibiotics are like pesticides to your "beehive" (your microbiome), wiping out your good bacteria with the bad.

Following the Johns Hopkins Protocol, I use herbal supplements and follow the recommended dosage for thirty days, then reassess. Patients with severe bloating sometimes require two to six months of a tailored program in order to eradicate the overgrowth of the bacteria causing their bloating. The protocol is as follows:

Original John Hopkins Protocol: 2 capsules twice daily of the following commercial herbal preparations: Dysbiocide and FC Cidal (Biotics Research Laboratories, Rosenberg, Texas) or Candibactin-AR and Candibactin-BR (Metagenics, Inc, Aliso Viejo, California) for 4 consecutive weeks.

Dr. de Mello's version of the protocol combined the following: 2 capsules each, 2 times a day before a meal for 8 weeks of the following: FC Cidal, Dysbiocide and Candibactin-AR.

In addition, we often recommend allicin (the active compound produced when garlic is crushed), oregano oil, berberine, our *GI Align* Product and our *Vital AM* to help with elimination.

PART IV: Antibiotics vs. Enzyme Treatments

The use of antibiotics has been proven ineffective in the treatment of biofilms because the associated symptoms tend to rebound, given the ability of the bacteria to use its biofilm in resisting the antibiotics.[31] Instead, I recommend using enzymes such as *nattokinase* and *lumbrokinase*, which are widely used in naturopathic and integrative medicine as biofilm disruptor, as the first step.

Lumbrokinase: Known in Chinese medicine as *di long*, meaning "earth dragon," this enzyme is derived from *Lumbricus rubellus*, or earthworms. It has been shown to promote the breakdown of fibrinogen, a protein involved in blood clotting. Earthworms

have been used for centuries in Traditional Chinese Medicine (TCM) to treat circulatory, lung, liver, and spleen disorders.
Dose: ranges from 20 milligrams (mg) to 40 mg, depending on the brand. I recommend starting with 20 mg and slowly moving up to 40 mg if your system can tolerate it.

Nattokinase: an enzyme extracted and highly purified from a traditional Japanese food called natto. It is a fermented, cheese-like food that has been used in Japan for many centuries as a folk remedy for heart and vascular diseases, as well as for its popular taste. Natto, an enzyme extracted from boiled soybeans that have been fermented with bacteria, is believed to work by thinning the blood to help break up blood clots.
Dose: 100 mg up to three times a day. Again, I strongly recommend discussing a regimen with your integrative practitioner or doctor and, if appropriate for you, to start slowly. Use one capsule of 100 mg a day and slowly move up to two times a day or more depending on the individual case and the recommendations from your practitioner.

N-acetyl cysteine or **NAC:** a powerful molecule that works against biofilms. It is a precursor of the "scavenger" amino acid antioxidant glutathione that has also proven effective against biofilms in chronic respiratory infections, for example.[32]

Additional Correcting Supplements
SAMe supplements, Omega 3s, olive oil and coconut oil, and betaine all help augment the methylation pathway. However, some of these compounds, especially SAMe, may actually make things worse in some people. The only way to know is to try it under the supervision of your integrative practitioner.

Other things we might try:

• Vitamins C, D, E, and probiotics
• Turmeric, raw garlic and raw onions (sources of glutathione)

- SAMe 400mg, 1,200–1,600 mg a day
- Omega 3: 1 (EPA/DHA) twice a day
- Methyl B12 shot, or sublingual, or nasal spray
- Curcumin, riboflavin B2
- Coconut oil: contains Lauricidin, a natural surfactant that helps inhibit the development of biofilms[33]
- Colloidal silver, which has also proven effective against biofilms to prevent wound infections
- Avoid medications that block B12 absorption, like proton pump inhibitors or antacids (Prilosec®, Prevacid®, Tums®)

Things Everyone Can Do (*In case you missed it*)
- **Avoid processed foods:** especially those that have added synthetic folic acid. Instead, eat whole foods with no added chemicals/preservatives.
- **Eat leafy greens:** (e.g., spinach, kale, chard, arugula) that are rich in folate.
- **Avoid taking meds that deplete or block folic acid,** like birth control pills with methotrexate.
- **Remove mercury amalgam fillings** with a trained biologic dentist.
- **Avoid toxic exposure:** eat grass fed, organic meat, and non-GMO vegetables
- **Avoid heavy metal exposure**
- **Gentle detox** twice a week. Try infrared saunas and epsom salt baths.
- **Exercise** with sweating

PART V: Diagnosis and Lab Testing

Diagnosis

Although bloating can cause significant patient distress, fortunately in most cases it is not a life-threatening condition. But even when only occasional bloating is present, it is a major inconvenience for millions and millions of individuals world-wide. I recommend that the evaluation of a patient includes:

- A carefully detailed history and physical examination to rule out any medical disorder as the cause of bloating.
- Specifically asking a patient if they have a history of anemia and/or unintentional weight loss. These symptoms may be a sign of malabsorption.
- A complete blood count, chemistry panel, including heavy metals, celiac sprue serology, and testing for Vitamins D and B12 levels, as this can also indicate malabsorption due to a genetic mutation, and a food sensitivity test.
- Hormone and thyroid panels, stool test to assess the microbiome and a breath test to rule out SIBO and H. pylori, bacteria known to cause GI ulcers.
- Imaging studies such as X-rays, ultrasound, MRI, and CT scans are not essential in the diagnosis of bloating, other than being helpful in ruling out GI obstruction, unless symptoms persist after initial treatment.

Laboratory Testing

Bloating and distension are tell-tale signs of bacterial over-growth. Although there is not a specific diagnostic test designed just for bloating or distention, a number of laboratory exams can help identify probable medical causes and rule out various associated disorders, such as SIBO. These include:

Stool analysis: A stool sample can be checked for the presence of blood or parasites, which can indicate infection. Further, this examination can rule out infection by *Yersinia, salmonella,* and/or *Campylobacter* organisms.

Lactose Intolerance Tests: If you're unable to digest dairy products, you may experience symptoms similar to IBS, like abdominal bloating, gas, and diarrhea. Lactose intolerance can be diagnosed through a breath test or by eliminating dairy products from your diet for several weeks and monitoring your results.

Blood workup: Many conditions can be confirmed by testing the blood for numerous substances and properties. There are hundreds of different types of blood tests that can be used to rule out several conditions that can lead to bloating. A full blood count is needed to rule out anemia, inflammation, or any electrolyte abnormality such as dehydration.

Lower GI Series (also known as the Small Bowel Follow-Through Test): A doctor uses an x-ray of your intestines to check for possible blockages. Before the test, your doctor will insert barium into your intestines through a tube in your anus. Barium is a liquid that makes the intestines more visible on the x-ray. The barium will highlight abnormalities in the esophagus and stomach. You're usually required to undergo a liquid diet and enema before the examination. A sedative can help you relax during the procedure. You may have some discomfort and discolored stools for a day or two after this exam.

An Upper GI Series such as the endoscopic procedure is used to diagnose stomach cancer, peptic ulcers, gastritis, reflux esophagitis, colon cancer, and diverticulitis.

Flexible Sigmoidoscopy or Colonoscopy (w/biopsy): These tests allow your doctor to view your rectum and colon with a small camera attached to a thin tube. The tube is gently inserted into your anus. As with the lower GI series test, this test usually requires a liquid diet and enema before examination. Taking a sedative may also be an option. Your doctor may recommend a colonoscopy to rule out the possibility of colon cancer if you fall into a certain risk group based on age, race, or family history.

CT Scan: Scanning of your pelvic region can rule out other possible causes of bloating discomfort, such as pancreatic or gallbladder problems.

Radiographic investigations: X-rays, depending on the location of the mass and associated symptoms

Chest x-ray: an x-ray of the structures inside the chest. A chest x-ray can illuminate physical abnormalities that could be causing a protrusion.

Ultrasound of abdomen and/or pelvis: looks for gallstones, abdominal aneurysm, or ectopic pregnancy.

Nuclear scan of gallbladder: useful in detecting acute cholecystitis.

Gallium scan: used to detect a diverticular abscess; a test that uses radioactive material (gallium) to search for the sources of infection in the body. In some cases, I also order an x-ray to rule out pneumonia.

Electrolyte tests: Electrolytes are essential substances in the human body that are vital for maintaining a healthy balance of water and acid-alkali. They are also important for ensuring normal muscle contractions and the transmission of nerve messages. Electrolytes are available in a large variety of foods.

Pancreatic enzyme test: This is a blood test to detect the presence of enzymes produced by the pancreas. Pancreatic enzymes include amylase, trypsin, and lipase. Pancreatic enzymes help us to digest carbohydrates, proteins, and fats in the duodenum of the small intestine. Medical conditions that can afflict the pancreatic enzymes include cystic fibrosis, pancreatic cancer, and pancreatitis.

Pregnancy test: This must also be ordered in all heterosexually active women of reproductive age that are experiencing bloating.

It is important to use tests to gather as much information as is possible about what is going on inside our bodies and to consider each and every factor that could be contributing to any adverse condition.

PART VI: SIBO Treatment

Small intestinal bacterial overgrowth, or SIBO, refers to an increase in number and type of bacteria living in our colon. While some bacteria in the small intestine is normal and needed to optimize the breakdown and absorption of nutrients, the colon (large intestine), not the small intestine, is home to the highest concentration of bacteria.

Because the digestive system plays a vital role in protecting our system from harmful substances, the walls of the intestines act as barriers, controlling what can be transported into our bodies. When bacteria overpopulate the small intestine, it leads to an increase in intestinal permeability, a condition in which bacteria and toxins are able to pass through the intestinal wall into the bloodstream, causing widespread GI inflammation.

Tight junctions, small gaps in the intestinal wall, allow water and nutrients to pass through. When the tight junctions become loose, gut wall permeability is increased, which, in turn, allows bacteria and toxins into the bloodstream. Increased gut wall permeability is commonly referred to as leaky gut syndrome, as previously noted.

While SIBO symptoms can mimic those seen in IBS, bloating and increased gas production are the most common symptoms of SIBO. This is followed by decreased nutrient and vitamin malabsorption, such as B12 and iron, among others. Serotonin, the "feel good" hormone, is a brain chemical, ninety percent of which is estimated to be produced in the gut. An imbalance of serotonin contributes to mood changes, anxiety, and depression. Serotonin levels also have an effect on medical conditions ranging from irritable bowel syndrome to osteoporosis and cardiovascular disease.

How Do We Diagnose SIBO?

A breath SIBO test, used specifically for diagnosing Small Intestinal Bacterial Overgrowth, is based on the principle that bacteria produce Hydrogen (H_2) and Methane (CH_4) gas in response to non-absorbed carbohydrates in the intestinal tract. Hydrogen gas can then freely diffuse to the bloodstream, where it is exhaled by the patient. A carbohydrate load, typically lactulose or glucose, is administered to the patient, and exhaled breath gases are analyzed at routine intervals.

With lactulose, a normal response would be a sharp increase in breath H_2 (and/or CH_4) once the carbohydrate load passes through the ileocecal valve into the colon. In a normal small intestine, glucose should be fully absorbed prior to reaching the ileocecal valve; therefore, any peak in breath H_2 or CH_4 is indicative of SIBO.

Generally an increase in H_2 of 20 parts per million within 60–90 minutes is considered to be diagnostic of SIBO.

Prokinetic Agents

Used to improve bloating, nausea, vomiting, and constipation, prokinetics help control the acid reflux that follows by strengthening the LES, causing the stomach contents to empty faster.

I typically recommend prokinetics for gastroesophageal reflux disease (GERD), together with heartburn medications and, sometimes, known PPIs (Proton Pump Inhibitors).

However, prokinetics are not free of side effects and must be used with caution. I only recommend that they be used when all other natural approaches, such as ginger, dandelion root, and burdock root, referred to as herbal bitters, have failed.

Prokinetic drugs work by increasing the strength of GI contractions, known as peristalsis, without disrupting the overall rhythm and function of the rest of the system. As we eat, swallowing induces primary peristalsis, moving the food down the esophagus and through the remainder of your digestive system.

PART VII: Take Control

Be aware of the potential causes of your bloating. There are many possible contributing factors to consider.

Check your diet: Certain foods such as broccoli, beans, onions, cabbage, cauliflower, brussels sprouts, lettuce, apples, pears, peaches, milk, chewing gum, carbonated drinks, and whole-grain foods can cause bloating. Bloating reduces if these specific foods are avoided.

Lactose Intolerance: the inability to digest lactose, a sugar present in milk and its products. It occurs when the small intestines fail to produce enough amounts of lactase, an enzyme needed for humans to properly digest the lactose. The symptoms of lactose intolerance include bloating, pain, stomach cramps, vomiting, and diarrhea following the intake of milk and milk products. Avoiding lactose-containing foods is recommended to prevent these types of discomfort.

Irritable Bowel Syndrome (IBS): a chronic functional gastrointestinal disorder. Patients with IBS may have abdominal pain, bloating, mucus in their stools, and diarrhea or constipation. In patients with IBS, avoiding foods that trigger their symptoms is recommended. Since there is a psychological aspect to IBS, patients may benefit from techniques to reduce stress.

Intestinal Obstruction: a condition where there is a blockage in the lumen of the intestines, preventing the flow of the abdominal contents. Causes of intestinal obstruction include roundworms, severe constipation, colon cancer, and intussusception (where one part of the intestine telescopes into another). The patient may present with pain in the abdomen, constipation, vomiting, abdominal distension, and bloating. Intestinal obstruction has to be managed immediately to prevent major complications.

Gastroparesis: a disorder where the movement of food is slowed down or stopped from the stomach to the intestine. This occurs due to damage to the vagus nerve that supplies the stomach muscle and causes it to contract. Diabetes neuropathy affecting the vagus nerve is a common cause of gastroparesis. Bloating is present in these patients.

Chronic Constipation: In patients suffering with this condition, bloating may be present due to the retention of stool in the large intestine, which is fermented by bacteria to release gas.

Celiac Disease: an autoimmune disease of the intestine with a genetic predisposition. Patients with celiac disease cannot digest gluten, a protein present in foods made of grains like wheat, barley, and rye. Consuming gluten causes various gastrointestinal symptoms including bloating. Patients should be put on a strict dietary restriction of gluten.

Cirrhosis of the Liver: a condition where the function of the liver deteriorates due to chronic liver disease and alcoholism. Bloating is seen in these patients due to the accumulation of fluid in the abdomen, a condition called ascites. The patients usually present with a history of an underlying liver disease.

Congestive Heart Failure: a condition where the pumping action of the heart is not as strong as it should be. Bloating in these patients is due to the accumulation of fluid in the abdomen, which may occur at a later stage. The patient often shows other signs of heart failure such as swelling of feet and shortness of breath.

Pancreatic Insufficiency: The pancreas secretes digestive enzymes. In patients with pancreatic insufficiency, the enzymes produced are not sufficient for the digestion of the food. These patients present with pain in the abdomen, bloating, and oily stools.

Kidney Disease: can lead to kidney failure, which causes fluid retention in the abdomen, leading to bloating.

Pregnancy: Increased levels of progesterone during early pregnancy leads to the relaxation of the intestine, which in turn can result in bloating.

Hypothyroidism: a decreased level of thyroid hormones. In patients with this condition, constipation and bloating are common due to the slow gut movement. Hypothyroidism is diagnosed through blood tests.

Babies and bloating: Newborns and infants often have a problem with bloating since they swallow a lot of air while suckling. Proper feeding technique and burping are necessary to prevent gas in babies.

Premenstrual Syndrome: experienced due to the hormonal variations for one or two weeks just before menstruation. The bloating is due to high estrogen levels leading to water retention. The bloating decreases after menstruation.

Surgical Interventions: Bloating presents in patients who have had recent gastric surgeries, due to gas accumulation in the stomach. Fundoplication, gastric banding, and other bariatric procedures can also cause bloating.

Parasites: Parasites, like Giardia, can cause bloating, watery diarrhea, and abdominal cramps. This problem can be diagnosed through repeated stool tests.

Malignancies: Cancers of the stomach, intestine, and ovaries can cause bloating. These conditions need to be ruled out in patients complaining of persistent bloating.

Increased Gas Production: Several studies using various techniques have not been able to show significant differences in gas production between "normal" volunteers and those with bloating.[34,35,36,37,38] In addition, even infusions of large amounts of gas (2,160 ml) into the intestinal tract of normal volunteers produced only a small change (less than 2 cm) in abdominal girth.

Impaired Gas Transit: Over twenty years ago, researchers demonstrated that some patients with bloating have abnormalities in intestinal transit, which could contribute to their symptoms.[39,40] Bloating correlates with gas retention in these patients.

Impaired Evacuation: Some patients cannot effectively evacuate gas, resulting in prolonged intestinal gas retention and symptoms of bloating and pain. Patients with functional bloating and constipation are less able to effectively evacuate infused gas and are much more likely to develop symptoms of abdominal distention.[41,42,43,44,45] Some of these patients appear to have a deficiency in the normal rectal reflex involved in intestinal gas propulsion.[46]

Abnormal Abdominal-Diaphragmatic Reflexes: Over sixty years ago, the possibility of an abnormal abdominal wall reflex, leading to bloating, was investigated.[47] In healthy adults, intestinal gas infusion *increases muscle activity* in the abdominal wall.[48] Gas infusion in bloated patients leads to *decreased* contraction of the abdominal wall muscles. This abnormal viscero-somatic reflex activity in patients with bloating means that abdominal wall muscles relax, rather than contract, with gaseous distention of the GI tract, emphasizing luminal gas.[49,50]

Abnormal Sensation or Perception: Patients with bloating are more sensitive to stretching and distention of the GI tract, compared to healthy individuals.[51,52] Healthy subjects generally tolerate intestinal gas quite a lot better because they propel and evacuate gas more efficiently.

Psychosocial Aspects: The prevalence and severity of bloating symptoms have been associated with decreased quality of life, and that psychosocial distress can contribute to the severity of a person's bloating.[53,54] As such, in order to be effective, any treatment strategy to eradicate bloating must address the psychological factors that are associated with it.

Gut Microflora: the bacteria that inhabit the intestinal tract (and their effects on both GI tract function and the body as a whole).

Approximately five hundred different species of bacteria reside within the colon, and microflora vary from one individual to another. Nearly all of these species are anaerobes (exist in the absence of oxygen). As discussed, gut bacteria imbalance leads to increased intestinal permeability, decreased immune response, and all kinds of damage to the microbiome.

Abnormalities in Posture: Some clinicians have reported that patients with significant complaints of bloating and abdominal distention appear to unconsciously change their body position, adopting a more lordotic (swayback) position. But no significant studies have found that patients with IBS appear to adopt a more lordotic position as compared to other patients.[55]

Normal Intestinal Gas: Colonic gas production is due *mostly* to the metabolism of food by colonic bacteria. Gas within the GI tract develops from several additional sources, including swallowing air, drinking carbonated beverages, or neutralization of acids and alkalis in the upper GI tract. For a number of reasons, it is difficult to define an *abnormal* amount of intestinal gas. No consensus has been reached on standardized definitions. In essence, bloating is primarily a sensory phenomenon that varies significantly from person to person, which makes the ability to accurately measure it in clinical practice very limited.

CHAPTER

10

Conclusion

*"Implementing new healthy habits in your life is not a
finish line to be crossed. It is a lifestyle to be lived."*
—E. de Mello, MD, PhD

Bloating and distension and an array of debilitating symptoms
that they cause are very common, yet poorly understood,
conditions. If you suffer from these symptoms, you should work
with your integrative practitioner to identify therapies that will
improve your specific symptoms.

Bloating is uncomfortable and can rob you of the quality of
life you used to enjoy. It leaves you feeling embarrassed, angry,
and confused about the next steps to take. No matter what steps
you may have taken to get rid of it, it sometimes rears its ugly
head at the most inopportune time. It is an invisible pain, and
most people will have no idea that you're suffering.

Affecting as many as 20–30 million Americans, bloating is
technically not a disease (as it does not permanently damage the
bowel); although in some cases, it may signal the beginning of
something more serious.

Initially, people suffering from increased gas, bloating,
abdominal pain, nausea, diarrhea, or constipation may brush off
these life-disrupting symptoms or rationalize it as "something I
ate" that will just pass. Unfortunately, if these symptoms persist,
they tend to get worse, leaving people feeling lost, embarrassed,

depressed, angry, and unattractive. My own medical practice, where a majority of patients with consistent bloating have SIBO, is evidence that this condition is on the rise. And because SIBO is not yet fully understood, it is often not recognized or is misdiagnosed.

Until now, it may have felt as though being bloated is something that you have just had to live with. You've tried everything!

Hopefully, after taking this journey with me, you understand that bloating is *not* some incurable mystery ailment that will wreak havoc on your life forever! Although there is no one-size-fits-all treatment, you should rest assured that it is more than possible to create an individualized plan that will relieve you of your bloating symptoms.

By better understanding your own amazing "beehive-like" structure—home to trillions of bacteria and other microorganisms—you can take back your life and *feel great* in your skin again.

Soon, the days where you felt out of control of your body will be long gone. It is time. Go for it!

About the Author

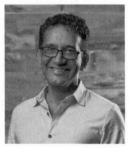

D R. **EDISON DE MELLO** is a Board Certified Integrative Physician and a licensed psychotherapist. The Founder and Medical Director of the Akasha Center in Santa Monica, he's treated patients from across the spectrum using his signature east-meets-west approach.

Born in Rio de Janeiro, Brazil, Dr. de Mello was introduced to the practice of integrative medicine by his beloved grandmother, Nana, at a very early age. Dr. de Mello remembers her as a natural healer who, with her many teas and potions, always had a remedy for the common everyday malady. Nana practiced her "medicine" with so much love and dedication that her simple presence, caring manner, smile, and unwavering respect for people were healing and inspiring. Nana's approach to healing and her loving mentorship were so profound for Dr. de Mello that a career in healthcare was a natural choice.

Envisioned as a "healing sanctuary," where all parts that compose a person, namely mind, body and spirit, are equally addressed when treating and preventing disease, The Akasha Center exemplifies Dr. de Mello's vision and strong commitment to the practice of integrative medicine. His goal is to help every patient get the best out of the integration of science-proven approaches to medicine, drawing from both the technological advances of the West and the ancient wisdom of the East.

Dr. de Mello is on the advisory board of several organizations such as Helpquide.org in Los Angeles, A.C.A.M. Midwifery Program in Guatemala (www.mayamidwifery.com), and the Sun Ray Peace and Meditation Society in Vermont (www.sun-ray.org). He is a member of the Academy of Integrative Health and Medicine (AIHM), The Institute of Functional Medicine (IMF), The American Academy of Family Physicians (AAFP), The American Association of Integrative Medicine, and Physicians for Social Responsibility.

He writes for a variety of publications and is a frequent guest on integrative medicine podcasts. He believes physicians should always *Meet their Patient before Meeting their Dis-EASE*, a belief that he puts into practice every day.

Endnotes / References

Chapter 1: When Bloating Is a Constant, Uninvited, Annoying Companion

1. Thiwan, S. (n.d.). Abdominal Bloating: A Mysterious Symptom. *UNC Center for Functional GI & Motility Disorders*, 4.

2. Levy, J. (2015, November 20). *Always Have A Bloated Stomach? Here Are 10 Reasons Why*. Dr. Axe. https://draxe.com/health/bloated-stomach/

3. Ibid

4. Ibid

5. Ibid

Chapter 2: Bacteria: Friend or Foe?

1. Chin-Lee, B., Curry, W. J., Fetterman, J., Graybill, M. A., & Karpa, K. (2014). Patient experience and use of probiotics in community-based health care settings. *Patient Preference and Adherence, 8*, 1513–1520. https://doi.org/10.2147/PPA.S72276

2. Shahbamdeh, M. (2019, September 6). *Probiotics: Market value in the United States, 2014–2024*. Statista. Retrieved

August 19, 2020, from https://www.statista.com/
statistics/994912/dollar-sales-probiotic-united-states/

3. Alcock, J., Maley, C. C., & Aktipis, C. A. (2014). Is eating
behavior manipulated by the gastrointestinal microbiota?
Evolutionary pressures and potential mechanisms. *Bioessays*,
36(10), 940–949. https://doi.org/10.1002/bies.201400071

4. *Humans Have Ten Times More Bacteria Than Human Cells: How
Do Microbial Communities Affect Human Health?* (2008, June 5)
ScienceDaily. Retrieved February 5, 2020, from https://
www.sciencedaily.com/releases/2008/06/080603085914
.htm

5. Kolata, G. (2012, June 13). In Good Health? Thank Your
100 Trillion Bacteria. *The New York Times*. https://www.
nytimes.com/2012/06/14/health/human-microbiome-
project-decodes-our-100-trillion-good-bacteria.html

6. Wenner, M. (2007, November 30). *Humans Carry More
Bacterial Cells than Human Ones*. Scientific American.
Retrieved February 5, 2020, from https://www.
scientificamerican.com/article/strange-but-true-humans-
carry-more-bacterial-cells-than-human-ones/

7. Steenbergen, L., Sellaro, R., van Hemert, S., Bosch, J. A.,
& Colzato, L. S. (2015). A randomized controlled trial
to test the effect of multispecies probiotics on cognitive
reactivity to sad mood. *Brain, Behavior, and Immunity*, *48*,
258–264. https://doi.org/10.1016/j.bbi.2015.04.003

Chapter 3: The Amazing Gut: A Beehive-like System

1. Founder, D. E. G. (2016, December 22). *Gut Health 101:
What Is the Microbiome?* Dr. Group's Healthy Living Articles.
https://www.globalhealingcenter.com/natural-health/
what-is-the-microbiome/

2. Ibid

3. Ishige, T., Honda, K., & Shimizu, S. (2005). Whole organism biocatalysis. *Current Opinion in Chemical Biology*, *9*(2), 174–180. https://doi.org/10.1016/j.cbpa.2005.02.001

4. Bianconi, E., Piovesan, A., Facchin, F., Beraudi, A., Casadei, R., Frabetti, F., Vitale, L., Pelleri, M. C., Tassani, S., Piva, F., Perez-Amodio, S., Strippoli, P., & Canaider, S. (2013). An estimation of the number of cells in the human body. *Annals of Human Biology*, *40*(6), 463–471. https://doi.org/10.3109/03014460.2013.807878

5. Zimmer, C. (2013, October 23). *How Many Cells Are In Your Body?* National Geographic. https://www.national geographic.com/science/phenomena/2013/10/23/how-many-cells-are-in-your-body/

6. Kolata, G. (2012, June 13). In Good Health? Thank Your 100 Trillion Bacteria. *The New York Times*. https://www.nytimes.com/2012/06/14/health/human-microbiome-project-decodes-our-100-trillion-good-bacteria.html

7. Genevieve, J. *Study reveals connection between microbiome and autoimmune disorders*. (2017, October 23). The University of Calgary. http://www.ucalgary.ca/news/study-reveals-connection-between-microbiome-and-autoimmune-disorders

8. Dinan, T. G., & Cryan, J. F. (2017). The Microbiome-Gut-Brain Axis in Health and Disease. *Gastroenterology Clinics of North America*, *46*(1), 77–89. https://doi.org/10.1016/j.gtc.2016.09.007

9. Founder, D. E. G. (2016, December 22). *Gut Health 101: What Is the Microbiome?* Dr. Group's Healthy Living Articles. https://www.globalhealingcenter.com/natural-health/what-is-the-microbiome/

10. Ibid

11. Ibid

12. Ibid

13. Ibid

Chapter 4: Candida Overgrowth: Microbiome Gone Wrong

1. World Health Organization. (2018, February 5). *Antibiotic resistance.* https://www.who.int/news-room/fact-sheets/detail/antibiotic-resistance

2. Huffnagle, G. B., & Noverr, M. C. (2013). The emerging world of the fungal microbiome. *Trends in Microbiology, 21*(7), 334–341. https://doi.org/10.1016/j.tim.2013.04.002

3. Jamal, M., Ahmad, W., Andleeb, S., Jalil, F., Imran, M., Nawaz, M. A., Hussain, T., Ali, M., Rafiq, M., & Kamil, M. A. (2018). Bacterial biofilm and associated infections. *Journal of the Chinese Medical Association: JCMA, 81*(1), 7–11. https://doi.org/10.1016/j.jcma.2017.07.012

Chapter 5: Nutrition

1. *Foods That Cause Gas, Ranked (and What to Eat Instead).* (2018, July 10). Dave Asprey Blog. https://blog.daveasprey.com/foods-that-cause-gas/

2. Ibid

3. Ibid

4. Ibid

5. Dennett, C. (2018, November 6). Perspective | Fructans, not gluten, might cause wheat sensitivity. Here's what you need to know. *Washington Post.* https://www.washingtonpost.com/lifestyle/wellness/fructans-not-gluten-might-cause-

wheat-sensitivity-heres-what-you-need-to-know/2018/11/05/
fcee5f2c-dbb3-11e8-b3f0-62607289efee_story.html

6. *Foods That Cause Gas, Ranked (and What to Eat Instead)*. (2018, July 10). Dave Asprey Blog. https://blog.daveasprey.com/ foods-that-cause-gas/

7. Ibid

8. Kobylewski, S., & Jacobson, M. F. (2012). Toxicology of food dyes. *International Journal of Occupational and Environmental Health*, *18*(3), 220–246. https://doi.org/10.1179 /1077352512Z.00000000034

9. Ibid

Chapter 6: Food Labels: What to Consume

1. *World's Fattest Countries*. (2007, February 8). Forbes. Retrieved August 19, 2020, from https://www.forbes. com/2007/02/07/worlds-fattest-countries-forbeslife-cx_ ls_0208worldfat.html

2. Jacobs, A. (2018, February 7). In Sweeping War on Obesity, Chile Slays Tony the Tiger. *The New York Times*. https://www.nytimes.com/2018/02/07/health/obesity-chile-sugar-regulations.html

3. Union of Concerned Scientists. (2016, July 19). *Transparency in Food Labeling*. https://www.ucsusa.org/resources/ transparency-food-labeling

4. Comments on Food Labeling: Revision of the Nutrition and Supplement Facts Labels. Docket No. FDA-2012-N-1210. Comment ID No. FDA-2012-N-1210-0322. July 31. Washington, DC: US Food and Drug Administration

5. Morsel Law. (2017, October 27). *Nature valley sued for claiming its granola bars are natural*. http://morsellaw.com/2014/12/ 08/nature-valley-isnt-natural-anymore/

6. Telpner, M. (2014, April 28). *Food Irradiation: 5 Things You Need To Know*. Meghan Telpner. https://www. meghantelpner.com/blog/food-irradiation-5-things-you-need-to-know/

7. Kittredge, Jack. (2013). The FDA—Aiming at Molehills While Ignoring Mountains? *The Natural Farmer.*

8. Mills, S. (1987). *Issues in food irradiation*. Science Council of Canada.

Chapter 7: The Three Amigos: Our Three Brains

1. Heart-Math Institute. (n.d.). *Science of the Heart: Exploring the Role of the Heart in Human Performance*. Retrieved February 23, 2020, from https://www.heartmath.org/research/science-of-the-heart/heart-brain-communication/

Chapter 8: Metabolism, Blood Flow, Sex, and Hormones

1. Morrison, John H., Brinton, Roberta D., Schmidt, Peter J., Gore, Andrea C. Estrogen, Menopause, and the Aging Brain: How basic Neuroscience Can Inform Hormone Therapy in Women. *Journal of Neuroscience.* 11 October 2006.

2. Hara, Yuko, Waters, Elizabeth M., McEwen, Bruce S., Morrison, John H. Estrogen Effects on Cognitive and Synaptic Health Over the Lifecourse. *Physiological Reviews.* 2015 June 24.

3. Stachenfeld, N. S. (2008). Sex Hormone Effects on Body Fluid Regulation. *Exercise and Sport Sciences Reviews*, 36(3), 152–159. https://doi.org/10.1097/JES.0b013e31817 be928

4. Selye, H., & Bassett, L. (1940). Diuretic Effect of Progesterone. *Proceedings of the Society for Experimental Biology*

and Medicine, 44(2), 502–504. https://doi.org/10.3181/
00379727-44-11508

5. American Urological Association. What is Low
Testosterone? https://www.urologyhealth.org/urologic-
conditions/low-testosterone?article=132

6. Nichols, Trent W., Faass, Nancy. *Optimal Digestive Health.*
Simon and Schuster. 22 Feb 2005.

7. BodyLogicMD. Bioidentical Hormones and Bloating—
How They Can Help. https://www.bodylogicmd.com/
for-women/bioidentical-hormones-and-bloating

8. McCormick, Kathleen. Digesting it All! https://www.
womensinternational.com/portfolio-items/digestion/

9. Sugaya, N, et al. Adrenal hormone response and
psychophysiological correlates under psychosocial stress in
individuals with irritable bowel syndrome. International
Journal of Psychophysiology. April 2012.

Chapter 9: Treatment Approaches

1. Mattar, R., de Campos Mazo, D. F., & Carrilho, F. J.
(2012). Lactose intolerance: Diagnosis, genetic, and clinical
factors. *Clinical and Experimental Gastroenterology, 5,* 113–121.
https://doi.org/10.2147/CEG.S32368

2. Ibid

3. Chan, A. O. O., Leung, G., Tong, T., & Wong, N. Y.
(2007). Increasing dietary fiber intake in terms of kiwifruit
improves constipation in Chinese patients. *World Journal
of Gastroenterology : WJG, 13*(35), 4771–4775. https://doi.
org/10.3748/wjg.v13.i35.4771

4. Odes, H. S., & Madar, Z. (1991). A double-blind trial of
a celandin, aloevera and psyllium laxative preparation in

adult patients with constipation. *Digestion*, *49*(2), 65–71. https://doi.org/10.1159/000200705

5. Sturtzel, B., Mikulits, C., Gisinger, C., & Elmadfa, I. (2009). Use of fiber instead of laxative treatment in a geriatric hospital to improve the wellbeing of seniors. *The Journal of Nutrition, Health & Aging*, *13*(2), 136–139. https://doi.org/10.1007/s12603-009-0020-2

6. Attaluri, A., Donahoe, R., Valestin, J., Brown, K., & Rao, S. S. C. (2011). Randomized clinical trial: Dried plums (prunes) vs. psyllium for constipation. *Alimentary Pharmacology & Therapeutics*, *33*(7), 822–828. https://doi.org/10.1111/j.1365-2036.2011.04594.x

7. Musso, G., Gambino, R., & Cassader, M. (2011). Interactions between gut microbiota and host metabolism predisposing to obesity and diabetes. *Annual Review of Medicine*, *62*, 361–380. https://doi.org/10.1146/annurev-med-012510-175505

8. Tremaroli, V., & Bäckhed, F. (2012). Functional interactions between the gut microbiota and host metabolism. *Nature*, *489*(7415), 242–249. https://doi.org/10.1038/nature11552

9. Quigley, E. M. M. (2010). Prebiotics and probiotics; modifying and mining the microbiota. *Pharmacological Research*, *61*(3), 213–218. https://doi.org/10.1016/j.phrs.2010.01.004

10. Pimentel M, Park S, Mirocha J, Kane SV, Kong Y. The effect of a non-absorbed oral antibiotic (Rifaximin) on the symptoms of the irritable bowel syndrome: a randomized trial. *Ann Intern Med.* 2006;145:557–563.

11. Sharara AI, Aoun E, Abdul-Baki H, Mounzer R, Sidani S, Elhajj I. A randomized double-blind placebo-controlled trial of rifaximin in patients with abdominal bloating and flatulence. *Am J Gastroenterol.* 2006;101:326–333.

12. Krishna, S., Bustamante, L., Haynes, R. K., & Staines, H. M. (2008). Artemisinins: Their growing importance in medicine. *Trends in Pharmacological Sciences, 29*(10), 520–527. https://doi.org/10.1016/j.tips.2008.07.004

13. Giacosa, A., Morazzoni, P., Bombardelli, E., Riva, A., Bianchi Porro, G., & Rondanelli, M. (2015). Can nausea and vomiting be treated with ginger extract? *European Review for Medical and Pharmacological Sciences, 19*(7), 1291–1296.

14. Badgujar, S. B., Patel, V. V., & Bandivdekar, A. H. (2014). Foeniculum vulgare Mill: A review of its botany, phytochemistry, pharmacology, contemporary application, and toxicology. *BioMed Research International, 2014,* 842674. https://doi.org/10.1155/2014/842674

15. Bub, S., Brinckmann, J., Cicconetti, G., & Valentine, B. (2006). Efficacy of an herbal dietary supplement (Smooth Move) in the management of constipation in nursing home residents: A randomized, double-blind, placebo-controlled study. *Journal of the American Medical Directors Association, 7*(9), 556–561. https://doi.org/10.1016/j.jamda.2006.06.001

16. Mirzaee, F., Hosseini, A., Jouybari, H. B., Davoodi, A., & Azadbakht, M. (2017). Medicinal, biological and phytochemical properties of Gentiana species. *Journal of Traditional and Complementary Medicine, 7*(4), 400–408. https://doi.org/10.1016/j.jtcme.2016.12.013

17. Chang, S.-M., & Chen, C.-H. (2016). Effects of an intervention with drinking chamomile tea on sleep quality and depression in sleep disturbed postnatal women: A randomized controlled trial. *Journal of Advanced Nursing, 72*(2), 306–315. https://doi.org/10.1111/jan.12836

18. Srivastava, J. K., Shankar, E., & Gupta, S. (2010). Chamomile: A herbal medicine of the past with bright

future. *Molecular Medicine Reports, 3*(6), 895–901. https://doi.org/10.3892/mmr.2010.377

19. Rahimi, R., & Abdollahi, M. (2012). Herbal medicines for the management of irritable bowel syndrome: A comprehensive review. *World Journal of Gastroenterology, 18*(7), 589–600. https://doi.org/10.3748/wjg.v18.i7.589

20. Allam, S., Krueger, D., Demir, I. E., Ceyhan, G., Zeller, F., & Schemann, M. (2015). Extracts from peppermint leaves, lemon balm leaves and in particular angelica roots mimic the pro-secretory action of the herbal preparation STW 5 in the human intestine. *Phytomedicine: International Journal of Phytotherapy and Phytopharmacology, 22*(12), 1063–1070. https://doi.org/10.1016/j.phymed.2015.08.008

21. Larijani, B., Esfahani, M. M., Moghimi, M., Shams Ardakani, M. R., Keshavarz, M., Kordafshari, G., Nazem, E., Hasani Ranjbar, S., Mohammadi Kenari, H., & Zargaran, A. (2016). Prevention and Treatment of Flatulence From a Traditional Persian Medicine Perspective. *Iranian Red Crescent Medical Journal, 18*(4). https://doi.org/10.5812/ircmj.23664

22. *Spices, oregano, dried Nutrition Facts & Calories.* (n.d.). Retrieved February 23, 2020, from https://nutritiondata.self.com/facts/spices-and-herbs/197/2

23. Ibid

24. Yang, J., Wang, H.-P., Zhou, L., & Xu, C.-F. (2012). Effect of dietary fiber on constipation: A meta analysis. *World Journal of Gastroenterology, 18*(48), 7378–7383. https://doi.org/10.3748/wjg.v18.i48.7378

25. Chambial, S., Dwivedi, S., Shukla, K. K., John, P. J., & Sharma, P. (2013). Vitamin C in Disease Prevention and Cure: An Overview. *Indian Journal of Clinical Biochemistry, 28*(4), 314–328. https://doi.org/10.1007/s12291-013-0375-3

26. Vermeer, C. (2012). Vitamin K: The effect on health beyond coagulation—an overview. *Food & Nutrition Research, 56.* https://doi.org/10.3402/fnr.v56i0.5329

27. Gil, M. I., Tomás-Barberán, F. A., Hess-Pierce, B., Holcroft, D. M., & Kader, A. A. (2000). Antioxidant activity of pomegranate juice and its relationship with phenolic composition and processing. *Journal of Agricultural and Food Chemistry, 48*(10), 4581–4589. https://doi.org/10.1021/jf000404a

28. Newman RA, Lansky EP, Block ML. Pomegranate: The Most Medicinal Fruit. Laguna Beach, California: Basic Health Publications; 2007. A Wealth of Phytochemicals; p. 120.

29. McKay, D. L., & Blumberg, J. B. (2006). A review of the bioactivity and potential health benefits of peppermint tea (Mentha piperita L.). *Phytotherapy Research: PTR, 20*(8), 619–633. https://doi.org/10.1002/ptr.1936

30. Chedid, V., Dhalla, S., Clarke, J. O., Roland, B. C., Dunbar, K. B., Koh, J., Justino, E., Tomakin, E., & Mullin, G. E. (2014). Herbal therapy is equivalent to rifaximin for the treatment of small intestinal bacterial overgrowth. *Global Advances in Health and Medicine, 3*(3), 16–24. https://doi.org/10.7453/gahmj.2014.019

31. von Rosenvinge, E. C., O'May, G. A., Macfarlane, S., Macfarlane, G. T., & Shirtliff, M. E. (2013). Microbial biofilms and gastrointestinal diseases. *Pathogens and Disease, 67*(1), 25–38. https://doi.org/10.1111/2049-632X.12020

32. Hogan, S., O'Gara, J. P., & O'Neill, E. (2018). Novel Treatment of Staphylococcus aureus Device-Related Infections Using Fibrinolytic Agents. *Antimicrobial Agents and Chemotherapy, 62*(2). https://doi.org/10.1128/AAC.02008-17

33. Ham, Y., & Kim, T.-J. (2016). Inhibitory activity of monoacylglycerols on biofilm formation in Aeromonas hydrophila, Streptococcus mutans, Xanthomonas oryzae, and Yersinia enterocolitica. *SpringerPlus*, *5*(1), 1526. https://doi.org/10.1186/s40064-016-3182-5

34. Lasser RB, Bond JH, Levitt MD. The role of intestinal gas in functional abdominal pain. *N Engl J Med*. 1975;293: 524–526.

35. Tomlin J, Lowis C, Read NW. Investigation of normal flatus production in healthy volunteers. *Gut*. 1991;32:665–669.

36. King TS, Elia M, Hunter JO. Abnormal colonic fermentation in irritable bowel syndrome. *Lancet*. 1998;352: 1187–1189.

37. Serra, J., Azpiroz, F., & Malagelada, J. R. (2001). Impaired transit and tolerance of intestinal gas in the irritable bowel syndrome. *Gut*, *48*(1), 14–19.

38. Caldarella MP, Serra J, Azpiroz F, Malagelada JR. Prokinetic effects in patients with intestinal gas retention. *Gastroenterology*. 2002;122:1748–1755.

39. Kellow JE, Phillips SF. Altered small bowel motility in irritable bowel syndrome is correlated with symptoms. *Gastroenterology*. 1987;92:1885–1893.

40. Kellow JE, Phillips SF, Miller LJ, Zinsmeister AR. Dysmotility of the small intestine in irritable bowel syndrome. *Gut*. 1988;29:1236–1243.

41. Serra J, Salvioli B, Azpiroz F, Malagelada JR. Lipid-induced intestinal gas retention in irritable bowel syndrome. *Gastroenterology*. 2002;123:700–706.

42. Caldarella MP, Serra J, Azpiroz F, Malagelada JR. Prokinetic effects in patients with intestinal gas retention. *Gastroenterology*. 2002;122:1748–1755.

43. Serra J, Azpiroz F, Malagelada JR. Mechanisms of intestinal gas retention in humans: impaired propulsion versus obstructed evacuation. *Am J Physiol Gastrointest Liver Physiol.* 2001;281:G138–G143.

44. Cann PA, Read NW, Brown C, Hobson N, Holdsworth CD. Irritable bowel syndrome: relationship of disorders in the transit of a single solid meal to symptom patterns. *Gut.* 1983;24:405–411.

45. Shim L, Prott G, Hansen RD, Simmons LE, Kellow JE, Malcolm A. Prolonged balloon expulsion is predictive of abdominal distension in bloating. *Am J Gastroenterol.* 2010;105:883–887.

46. Passos MC, Serra J, Azpiroz F, Tremolaterra F, Malagelada JR. Impaired reflex control of intestinal gas transit in patients with abdominal bloating. *Gut.* 2005;54:344–348.

47. Alvarez W. Hysterical type of nongaseous abdominal bloating. *Arch Intern Med.* 1949;84:217–245.

48. Tremolaterra F, Villoria A, Azpiroz F, Serra J, Aguadé S, Malagelada JR. Impaired viscerosomatic reflexes and abdominal-wall dystony associated with bloating. *Gastroenterology.* 2006;130:1062–1068.

49. Villoria A, Azpiroz F, Soldevilla A, Perez F, Malagelada JR. Abdominal accommodation: a coordinated adaptation of the abdominal wall to its content. *Am J Gastroenterol.* 2008;103:2807–2815.

50. Accarino A, Perez F, Azpiroz F, Quiroga S, Malagelada JR. Abdominal distention results from caudo-ventral redistribution of contents. *Gastroenterology.* 2009;136: 1544–1551.

51. Mertz H, Naliboff B, Munakata J, Niazi N, Mayer EA. Altered rectal perception is a biological marker of

patients with irritable bowel syndrome. *Gastroenterology.* 1995;109:40–52.

52. Bouin M, Plourde V, Boivin M, et al. Rectal distention testing in patients with irritable bowel syndrome: sensitivity, specificity, and predictive values of pain sensory thresholds. *Gastroenterology.* 2002;122:1771–1777.

53. Koloski NA, Talley NJ, Boyce PM. Does psychological distress modulate functional gastrointestinal symptoms and health care seeking? A prospective, community cohort study. *Am J Gastroenterol.* 2003;98:789–797.

54. Song JY, Merskey H, Sullivan S, Noh S. Anxiety and depression in patients with abdominal bloating. *Can J Psychiatry.* 1993;38:475–479.

55. Maxton DG, Martin DF, Whorwell PJ, Godfrey M. Abdominal distension in female patients with irritable bowel syndrome: exploration of possible mechanisms. *Gut.* 1991;32:662–664.

Glossary

Adrenal glands: endocrine glands that produce important hormones like epinephrine and norepinephrine, adrenaline, cortisol (the stress hormone), and even a small amount of testosterone.

Andropause: equivalent to a "male menopause"; age-related changes in male hormone levels, leading to a group of symptoms, among them testosterone deficiency, androgen deficiency, and late-onset hypogonadism.

Antibiotic resistance: bacteria that becomes resistant to antibiotics due to patients not taking the entire required dosage of antibiotics

Betaine: a crystalline compound with basic properties found in many plant juices.

Biofilm: a thin, slimy film of bacteria that adheres to a surface.

Bioidentical hormone replacement (BIHRT): man-made hormones that function the same as endogenous hormones—usually sex hormones like estrogen, progesterone, and testosterone.

Brain-gut axis: the powerful chemical connection between your gut and brain.

Candida: a type of yeast; a single-celled microorganism that grows in humans; overgrowth of candida is very common; growth can occur in the mouth, intestinal tract, skin, and genital area.

Casein: a milk-derived protein.

Celiac disease: an immune disease. People with this disease cannot consume gluten, which is found in foods like wheat, barley, and rye.

Chronic fatigue syndrome: a disorder characterized by extreme fatigue, lasting at least six months, which does not improve with rest.

Complementary medicine: treatment of a patient beyond scientific approaches; not supposed to replace scientific approach but can be practiced alongside it. Acupuncture, osteopathic medicine, massage, and herbal treatments are examples of complementary medical approaches.

Cortisol: a stress hormone released by adrenal glands; can lead to problems like high blood pressure if not managed

Distended: a bloated abdomen

Dysbiosis: microbial imbalance

Elimination diet: identifies which foods your GI system has difficulty tolerating.

Endocrinology: the field of study that explains how hormones work.

ENS (Enteric Nervous System): part of the autonomic nervous system that controls the gastrointestinal tract.

Estrobolome: refers to the specific set of bacterial genes that *code* for the enzymes that metabolize estrogen in our guts.

Estrogen: a sex hormone that is essential to women's reproductive development and maintenance. It plays a key role during puberty in the development of female secondary sexual characteristics; it also plays a role in restoring synaptic health and improving working memory.

Fight or flight: feeling the need to escape or fight when there's a threat. The brain turns on this survival mode and diverts attention away from proper digestion and elimination in order to conserve the energy needed to survive.

Flora: the microorganisms that live in our gut.

FODMAP diet: Fermentable Oligosaccharides, Disaccharides, Monosaccharides, and Polyols. These are poorly digested by the body, so a FODMAP diet avoids them. Examples of FODMAP food include wheat and other grains, fructose, dairy, and some legumes like beans.

Follicular phase: the preovulatory phase. During this phase, follicles stimulated by FSH and LH in the ovaries mature and estrogen production increases. Every menstrual cycle, only one follicle matures.

FSH: follicular-stimulating hormone; gonadotropin that stimulates the gonads—testes in males and ovaries in females

Gonads: organs where gametes are produced. In males, sperm are produced in the testes; in females, eggs are produced in the ovaries.

Gut epithelium: walls of the gut

GMO: genetically modified. This means that the whole food or ingredients used to make a particular product are altered at the genetic level by adding genetic material from different species or by making other changes that couldn't happen through traditional breeding.

Herxheimer reaction: also known as "die-off;" sudden increase in endotoxins (or bacterial waste) when bacteria and other microbes die; also a possible reaction to antifungals or antibiotics.

High fructose corn syrup: a sugar-based sweetener derived from corn syrup.

Hypothalamic-pituitary-adrenal (HPA) axis: made up of the hypothalamus, pituitary gland, and adrenal gland. The HPA axis regulates all hormone production in the body, including thyroid, adrenal, and sex hormones. It's extremely important when considering hormone imbalance issues.

IBS: irritable bowel syndrome; chronic; affects the large intestine

Immunocompromised: someone who has a weakened or impaired immune system; they are more affected by infections and diseases because their immune system has a harder time fighting them off

Intermittent fasting: a practice of meal timing in which one eats only during certain windows of time.

Invasive Candidiasis: a serious infection that can affect the blood, vital organs, and even your bones.

Johns Hopkins protocol: a method of treatment, dubbed by Dr. de Mello, in which one treats patients first with lifestyle changes before treating with medications. For example, life changes include diet, sleep, and exercise.

Leaky Gut: a condition in which the lining of the gut, specifically the pores, become inflamed and swollen. In turn, this allows the pores to expand. When this happens, the pores allow unfiltered and undigested large substances to pass through the bloodstream creating auto-immune inflammatory conditions and inflammatory response.

Leptin: a protein hormone produced by fat cells. One of leptin's jobs is to tell your brain to use the body's fat stores for energy.

LH: gonadotropin that stimulates the gonads—testes in males and ovaries in females

Luteal phase: The luteal phase begins soon after ovulation and lasts for two weeks. During this phase, the uterus's main job is to prepare for a possible pregnancy.

Lycasin: the trade name given by Roquette for hydrogenated glucose syrup. One of the major components of Lycasin is maltitol, derived from the hydrogenation of maltose.

Melatonin: a hormone that is produced in the stomach during meals as well as in the brain during sleep. Melatonin can help with bloating by regulating stomach acid while also increasing the production of an enzyme called pepsin, whose function is to move food from the stomach into the intestines.

Menopause: a period in a woman's life when her body has no more eggs to be released. Estrogen and progesterone levels stay low, and the endometrium starts to atrophy. It is often accompanied by symptoms like hot flashes, sweats, mood changes, and weight gain, among many others.

Menstruation: otherwise known as a woman's "period"; it begins at the onset of puberty and continues until menopause. Hormones signal for the shedding of the endometrial lining, and blood is expelled through the vagina

Monosaccharide: simple sugar-like glucose; cannot be broken down into smaller sugars

Mycotoxins: mold spores and mold metabolites that can also be present in the air, especially under very moist conditions. These spores, if inhaled, can negatively affect your immune system.

Candida overgrowth could occur which could product myco-toxins and make you feel horribly sick.

Naturopathic medicine: alternative form of medicine that uses natural and herbal treatments

Neurotransmitter: a chemical substance that is released at the end of a nerve fiber by the arrival of a nerve impulse and, by diffusing across the synapse or junction, causes the transfer of the impulse to another nerve fiber, a muscle fiber, or some other structure.

Neurohormones: chemical messenger molecules that are released in the blood system by neurons and are vital for development, growth, reproduction, feeding, and behavior.

Omega 3s: fatty acids that are essential nutrients; manage and lower the risk of heart problems

Ovaries: female gonads where eggs are produced

Ovulation: typically happens in the middle of the menstrual cycle, when an egg is expelled from the ovary into the fallopian tube

Preeclampsia: a condition in pregnant women indicated by high blood pressure, sometimes with fluid retention and an increased, dangerous level of protein in the urine.

PPI: proton-pump inhibitor; a group of medications whose main action is a pronounced and long-lasting reduction of stomach acid production. Within the class of medications, there is no clear evidence that one agent works better than another. They are the most potent inhibitors of acid secretion available.

Progesterone: a sex hormone that is crucial in maintainence of the uterus for pregnancy.

PMS: premenstrual syndrome; typically happens right before a woman's period, in which her mental and physical states are negatively affected; symptoms include mood swings, tender breasts, irritability, cramps, and fatigue, among many others; it can also cause bloating

rBGH: recombinant bovine growth hormone is used in cows. It mimics the natural bovine growth hormone found in cow's milk, which is consumed by humans; some speculate that there could be adverse effects on humans who drink milk made from cows who are treated with this hormone.

SAMe supplements: a correcting supplement; can treat a multitude of diseases, but may make some symptoms, like bloating, worse, so should only be used under recommendation of medical provider.

Scavenger antioxidant amino acid: molecules that inhibit free radical reactions to either delay or inhibit cellular damage.

Semi-dwarf wheat: wheat with its stem cut short, made for faster maturity, higher yield, and higher profit

Serotonin: neurotransmitter; mood regulator; also regulates appetite and digestion, along with sleep and memory. Some postulate that low levels of serotonin lead to depression.

SIBO: small intestinal bacterial overgrowth; affects the small intestine; occurs when bacteria that normally grow outside of the small intestine start to grow there; it causes uncomfortable symptoms like diarrhea, bloating, and pain.

SIBO breath test: shows how bacteria in the gut are functioning

Testosterone: hormone that is produced mainly by cells in the *gonads* in men (*ovaries* in women), with a small amount produced in the *adrenal glands* of both sexes; responsible for male secondary sex characteristics, regulates cortisol, aids in our mental, physical, and emotional health, increases and strengthens muscle mass, enhances sex drive.

Transceptors: a transporter-substrate complex that transduces signals to the inside of a cell.

Ulcerative colitis: an IBD that causes persistent sores, ulcers, and inflammation in the colon.

Vagus nerve: carries signals back and forth between the GI tract and the brain; in charge of parasympathetic control of digestion.

Made in the USA
Middletown, DE
26 October 2021